Hijacking the Brain

Hijacking the Brain

How Drug and Alcohol Addiction Hijacks Our Brains
The Science Behind Twelve-Step Recovery

Louis Teresi, MD

in collaboration with

Harry Haroutunian, MD

authorHOUSE®

AuthorHouse™
1663 Liberty Drive
Bloomington, IN 47403
www.authorhouse.com
Phone: 1-800-839-8640

Published by AuthorHouse   10/04/2011

ISBN: 978-1-4634-4484-6 (sc)
ISBN: 978-1-4634-4483-9 (hc)
ISBN: 978-1-4634-4485-3 (e)

Library of Congress Control Number: 2011913596

Contents

The Threat of Drug and Alcohol Addiction to Mankind ~ The Disease Model of Addiction ~ What Is a Disease? ~ What Are the Causes of Addiction and Alcoholism? ~ Genetic Predisposition ~ Psychological and Social Factors in the Etiology of Addiction ~ Stress as a Predominant Psychological Etiology ~ Comorbidity of Psychiatric Illness and Substance Abuse ~ What "Alterations in Known Body Systems" Are Caused by Addiction? ~ What Are the "Signs and Symptoms" of Addiction? ~ Institutional Adoption of the Disease Model of Addiction ~ Addictive Potential of Drugs and Alcohol ~ Having a Disease is NOT an Excuse ~ Robert H.: Chicken or the Egg

Possible Evolutionary Advantage of Drug Use By Ancient Man ~ Evolution of the Human Brain ~ The Evolutionary Advantage of Emotion ~ Emotions in Animals ~ Emotions in Humans ~ Plant-Derived Psychoactive Drugs ~ Psychoactive Drug Use in Animals ~ Psychoactive Drug Use in Ancient Cultures ~ Effect of Psychoactive Drugs on Emotions: Imaginary "Fitness" ~ John S.: Courage in a Bottle

Processing Emotions in Addiction - Is Cognitive Impairment Reversible?
- Neurogenesis and Neuroplasticity - Rewiring Brain Networks - Stress
Inhibits Neurogenesis - Summary

Jane S.: Experience, Strength, and Hope - About Twelve-Step Programs -
Why Anonymous? - A Physical, Mental and Spiritual Malady - Twelve-Step
Meetings and Sponsors - Effectiveness of Twelve-Step Programs - Taking
the Mystery Out of the Miracle of Twelve-Step Recovery - Working the
Twelve Steps: Reducing Fear, Anger, and Stress - Attitude of Gratitude

Carl L.: Chilling Out - Spiritual Principles and Beliefs - This Doctor's
Opinion: Spiritual Practices and Recovery - Meditation: Reducing
Emotional Distress - Meditation and the Brain - Effect of Prayer on
the Brain - Meditation and the Body: Reducing Stress - Meditation for
"Breaking" Habitual Behaviors - Mindfulness-Based Stress Reduction
Therapy for Sobriety

Joe M.: Almost "Going Out" - Groups and Recovery - What We Can
Learn from Animal Populations - The Rewarding Nature of Positive
Social Interaction - Oxytocin, the "Comfort" Hormone - Maternal
Bonding and Antistress Effects of Oxytocin - The Antistress Effects of
Oxytocin in Non-Mother-Infant Relations - The Prosocial Effects of
Oxytocin in Non-Mother-Infant Relations - Somatosensory Stimulation
and Oxytocin: The Massage Factor - The Physiology of Trust and Empathy
- Stress Promotes Social Interaction and Bonding: Seeking Comfort -
More Meetings = More Empathetic Social Support = Less Stress - Role of

the Therapy Dog ~ Comfort Music ~ Altruism and Recovery ~ Proof of the "Joy of Giving" ~ What Do Apes Have to Do with Recovery?

To my lovely and enduring wife, Amy
And the three gifts she gave me
Joseph, Giana, and Cara
&
To all who suffer from the incarceration of addiction
To those who love them
&
In respect for those who have been hurt by them

A percentage of royalties from the sale of this work are contributed to the
Betty Ford Foundation for the expressed purpose of funding scholarships for
those in need.

From the Lawyers

This publication contains the opinions and ideas solely of the author. It is intended to provide helpful and informative material on the subjects addressed in the publication. It is sold with idea that the author and publisher are not rendering medical, health, or any other kind of personal or professional services in the book.

The author and the publisher disclaim any representation of any Twelve-Step organization or their affiliates, or other health-care institutions. The author disclaims any formal association any specific addiction or alcohol treatment facility, nor does he endorse any specific facility.

In some circumstances, the scientific data in this book has been simplified to facilitate understanding of relatively complex neural and hormonal processes in the body.

The author and the publisher disclaim any liability, loss, or risk, personal or otherwise, which is incurred as a consequence, directly or indirectly, of the use and application of any of the contents of this book. Readers are advised to consult a license health care professional or other competent trusted advisor before adopting suggestions in this book.

Author's Note: My Perspective

At a young age, about fourteen, I made a commitment to my mother and myself that I was going to do something good for the planet. She raised me to be selfless, honest, and hard working. She raised me to be thankful to my creator. As a young man, I realized God was good to me. I had athletic ability and a reasonable mind. I wanted to thank Him by doing something for the rest of His creation. My mom raised me in the Catholic Church, although now I consider myself "Christian-lite." I believe in a loving God, Creator of all things, but I do not identify strongly with any particular religion. I think most, if not all, religions are good, as long as they teach principles of living that demonstrate respect and empathy for others and promote altruism. I believe that selfishness and arrogance are the root of all-evil.

Aristotle once said, *"I am man and nothing man shall be alien to me."* I liked that. As I matured, I realized I wanted to have a family and provide the best I could for them. Becoming a doctor seemed like a good fit for me. As a man, a doctor, and a good son, I can say that my intention in writing this book is to reach the addict, alcoholic, and their families, suffering with this dreaded disease, so that they may suffer no longer.

⌐

My perspective is that of a physician, biologist, and scientist, educated in traditional institutions with traditional scientific values. I practice evidenced-based medicine and, in twenty-four years of practice, have found that it works. My specialty, MR imaging, requires millimeter precision, so I am scrupulous. I have to be "right" better than 99 percent of the time, or I am out of a job. It is very stressful sometimes. (On a personal level, I can say that I am a perfectionist suffering from many flaws.) The diagnostic decisions I make are based upon seemingly endless scientific literature, which I study constantly. I applied this same traditional scientific rigor and precision to the study of materials covered in this book.

As a biologist, I believe all human behaviors have a motive, the motive is known only to the individual, and sometimes even the individual does not have rhetorical consciousness of their own motive; that is, they cannot put it into words. When I see a behavior in a person, I can only interpret it from my perspective, although I make every effort to take the perspective of others or no one, to respect scientific objectivity, and not to impart judgment.

For example, when I see an adult light a cigarette, I see a biological organism with a consciousness taking a substance known to make it feel good (nicotine) in a vehicle known to cause illness (smoke). The individual's motivation is likely "to feel better." Knowing from my own (former) experience with tobacco, a smoker generally *likes* a cigarette all the time, because nicotine is addictive and causes cravings, but smokers *really need* a cigarette when they are stressed; that is, the craving is magnified. Maybe the person lighting up is stressed. I do not know. I know that the nerve cells in the reward centers of the brain activated by the stimulant, nicotine, are intimately related to the nerve cells that perceive and process stress, so the statement "a stressed person lighting a cigarette" makes sense to me. I know that linking of the reward and stress centers in our brains is evolutionarily adaptive. I know that nicotine, as a stimulant, does not relieve stress like a sedative (e.g., Valium); we just think it can because it makes us feel better as a stimulant to our reward centers. This is my perspective.

The same interpretation could be said of other behaviors, like eating and sex. We like them anytime, but we really want them or need them when we're stressed. I "stress eat" all the time, usually on carrots and celery, but tortilla chips are better, and "Red Vine" licorices hit the bull's-eye on *my* reward centers. Nail biting and restless/bouncing legs or feet are also "nervous habits," with the only reward being that of discharging nervousness. This is my experience.

Through my studies in biology, I learned that, in many animals lower than man on the phylogenetic tree, there are numerous examples of animals exhibiting "displacement behaviors" when stressed to discharge the pent-up energy of stress. For example, when two male ducks come to the common boundary of their territories simultaneously, rather than engage in combat and risk possible injury, they furiously peck at the ground in "displaced" aggression. Male chimps, when quarantined from a potential female mate in heat, will eat voraciously, chew bark and bang their cages. The male wants to have sex with the female, but cannot, so he displaces his nervous energy, his stress, elsewhere. (I have been known to do the same.) Maybe the smoker is "displacing" some pent-up stress; maybe he just wants to feel good. I do not really know. My interpretation is dependent on my perspective as a biologist. Relevant to this book, chimps also use mood-altering substances.

In the text of this book, I will share with you many such examples from the animal kingdom, particularly mammals. *This is because all mammals have reward and limbic systems (centers of emotions, motivation and memory), as well as biological stress responses, virtually identical to man's. Animals, however, are easier to study because their behaviors are not confused by cultural, religious, or psychological influences.* My perspective is that of a comparative biologist, one who studies the similarities and differences amongst species. As all comparative biologists will tell you, our study is not so much about understanding those who share the planet with us *Homo sapiens*, however, more an opportunity to gain insight into the human condition uncomplicated by our religious, cultural and psychological nuances.

For example, I once heard a mental-health professional proclaim that addiction primarily was due to an individual being "hopeless and helplessness." I respect this perspective and believe that, in part, it is true. However, in my opinion, this explanation misses the target. It does not explain to me the multiple examples from the animal kingdom of animals using mood-altering substances, particularly, several strains of "addict rodents" that are referenced in this book. I believe that "hopelessness and helplessness" exacerbate addiction because of the *stress* associated with these states of mind. This is why, when you shock an alcoholic rodent's tail (i.e., stress it), the alcoholic rodent will drink more. The rodent is stressed, not "hopeless and helpless." I believe hopelessness and helplessness exacerbate addiction because they are cognitive and emotional states characterized by *stress*.

I also have the perspective of a recovering alcoholic. There were many fun drinking years—and too many bad. I knew I had an addiction to alcohol, and could not stop. At the time, I did not know why, although I believe I do now. A few days ago, my son, a handsome, intelligent eighteen year old, stepped into my home office while I was writing this book, stood next to my desk, and said: "It's the only thing you couldn't beat on your own: alcohol." I acknowledged him with a firm: "No doubt about it . . .

Kicked my ass. Plain and simple." My entire life I have worked very hard and have taken pride in excelling at whatever task I undertook. Being stubbornly self-sufficient, I never needed to ask for help in anything. I had very successful academic and medical careers. I ran marathons, was a decorated football player, won sailing regattas, published multiple scientific papers, lectured at scientific meetings, made a good living and raised loving family. (I have a long list of flaws, as well.) *Alcohol brought me to my knees; it almost killed me.* I now enjoy the gift of sobriety, but to get sober, for the first time in my life, I needed help. I found that help in a first class treatment center and the rooms of Alcoholics Anonymous.

When the treatment center doctor told me that I have an organic brain disease, alcoholism, and that the best-known "cure" was practicing a Twelve-Step program, I thought *he* was on drugs. My understanding at the time was that Twelve-Step programs invoked God and the solution to my alcoholism was a "spiritual awakening." I believe in God but am in no way religious, and a spiritual awakening was out of the question. The doctor showed me the studies proving that Twelve-Step programs work, if practiced enthusiastically; addicts and alcoholics achieve sobriety and improve their lives. He told me that the "spiritual solution" does not necessarily refer to God, but our relationships with others, nature, and ourselves. In fact, he said, I did do not have to believe in God at all to practice the Twelve Steps and achieve recovery.

I was intrigued, but the two dots—*(1) an organic brain disease and (2) a spiritual solution*—were too far apart for my scientific mind. I needed a solid scientific explanation for how a spiritual program can arrest an organic brain disease. Filled with the suspicions of a hard-core scientist, I embarked on a journey to connect the dots and explain to myself, in scientific terms, what happened to my brain and how the Twelve-Step programs could arrest it: I wrote *Hijacking the Brain*.

Hijacking the Brain interweaves themes from evolutionary biology, sociobiology, neuroscience, cognitive neuroscience, addiction medicine, and Twelve-Step programs to bring coherence and salience to our understanding of the neural and physiological bases of addiction and recovery. Recent rapid growth in the fields of neuroscience, neuroimaging and interpersonal neurobiology has given us new, dramatic insights into the neural and hormonal correlates of substance abuse and addiction. They also have afforded us an unprecedented look at the theoretical neural and physiologic bases of the success of Twelve-Step programs for recovery. Nothing in this book challenges the integrity of the Twelve Steps or Traditions of Twelve-Step fellowships. There is nothing in this book promoting God, or any particular religious belief. My personal views on God and religion are quite tolerant and centric, and referenced only lightly in the text. *The sole intention of Hijacking the Brain is to connect the dots between an "organic brain disease" and a "spiritual solution" with sound physical, scientific evidence.*

Several personal stories are presented to make palpable the conceptual themes. The personal stories in this publication are true, without modification or exaggeration; however, the names, professional associations, and other personal information have been changed in respect for these individuals' anonymity. These stories are representative of my own experience.

My story is not included, out of respect for all individuals involved as well as to protect my own anonymity and sobriety. Suffice it to say, I suffered many of the symptoms and consequences of a practicing alcoholic. There was some debate within my family and circle of friends about including my story. In this discussion, we recognized that *anonymity protects an individual from shame*, and there is shame in this culture for having the disease of alcoholism or addiction. We are considered by some to be weak, undisciplined or of lower moral standards. I am none of these, nor are most, if not all, of my friends with this disease. Certainly, some of the behaviors of the alcoholic and addict are deplorable and shameful, as they should be, but having a disease is not. I am ashamed of some of my behaviors while under the influence, however, I am *not* ashamed of having the disease of alcoholism. Shame and its incumbent stress only fuel the disease. For this reason alone, my story will remain within my inner circle. (The relationship of *stress and addiction* are addressed in Chapter 5; *shame* in Chapters 2, 9, and especially 7; and *anonymity* in Chapter 9.)

I wrote the text for the lay audience, at the level of a *Scientific American* or *Discover* article, avoiding as much as possible the scientific language that can wear a reader down. I admit some of the anatomy and physiology in Chapters 3 and 4 are tedious; however, I have thrown in ample illustrations of neural pathways, anatomy, and various biological relationships and interactions to facilitate the reader's progress. For those not interested in the neurobiology, you may skip Chapters 3 and 4 entirely. Skimming the text and looking at the pictures may suffice in these chapters. I do it all the time when weary. *Remember, however, the brain is what we are, and having an understanding of its workings can only help, particularly in the case of addiction, an organic brain disease.*

Hijacking the Brain is divided into two books: Book I addresses the *problem* and Book II, the *solution.* In Book I, we review the definition of a disease, the evolution of addiction and the brain, the neuroscience of cravings and dependency, the role of stress in addiction, and addiction-related cognitive impairment. In Book II we look at the scientific explanation for the success of Twelve-Step recovery programs, the role of meditation in sobriety, and the value of social (group) empathy in recovery. *Important subject matter is italicized* and there are several illustrations to facilitate skimming the text. I found the material to be fascinating, absolutely fascinating. I trust you will, too. *Enjoy the read!*

Introduction:

Unlocking the Mystery of the Miracle of Recovery

Addictive mind-altering drugs and alcohol are the bane and burden of civilized mankind, negatively altering the lives and even killing, directly or indirectly, millions of human beings throughout history. Every year many of us *Homo sapiens*, even those well educated and/or financially successful, find ourselves in jail, losing a job or a family, or even killing another human being as a consequence of our alcohol or drug addiction. The cost of addiction to our society is enormous. Why are human beings vulnerable and willing prey to the effects of mind-altering substances? Why do human beings take addictive mind-altering substances despite substantial and often horrific negative consequences, such as the loss of family, a job, and a reputation or legal or psychiatric incarceration? Why do some alcoholics and addicts literally drink or drug themselves to death?

Most addicts and alcoholics start using mood-altering substances in response to life stress: the loss of a loved one, financial distress, fear of failure, etc. The negative emotions associated with life stresses are essentially fear, resentment, and sorrow. These emotions and the horrible feeling of stress in our lives can be placated by drugs and alcohol. We primarily seek drugs and alcohol to dampen our negative thoughts and make us feel better. While intoxicated, one could say we have a false sense of Darwinian fitness. We feel stronger, until the mood-altering substance wears off and life's hard reality comes into focus again.

What is the current neuroscience behind how drugs and alcohol make us feel better? Although different classes of drugs affect different areas of the brain, the vast majority of recreational drugs stimulate the one common denominator in our central nervous system—the *"seat of our soul,"* if you will—the primitive reward centers of the brain. This part of our brain is called the *limbic system.*

The limbic system is our primitive brain, and evolved over millions of years to ensure our survival—that is, until mood-altering drugs and alcohol were introduced to mankind. *The limbic reward centers are the origins of emotion, memory, and motivation.* Just like good food or sex, a promotion at work, or winning the lottery make us feel good, a sip of a drink or a hit of a mood-altering drug affect the same "feel-good" center in our brains. By stimulating our limbic reward system, drinking and drugging make us feel good; it is that simple. *The limbic system is deep in our midbrain and virtually inaccessible to our conscious thoughts.* We have difficulty finding the exact words to describe the euphoria we experience during heightened limbic activity, as well as the cravings we suffer when these reward centers are deprived.

Proper functioning of our reward centers ensures the survival of our species. It has been said that individuals of our species have three basic instincts: (1) security (food and shelter), (2) reproduction, and (3) socialization. In the absence of mind-altering substances, our brains work wonderfully in the pursuit of instincts. We find food to eat and water to drink, build homes to protect our bodies, enter into relationships to reproduce, and develop social networks to ensure that the needs of instincts 1 and 2 are met, as well as to diversify the genetic pool. These instincts are hard-wired into the deep-seated reward centers of our brain, which command our higher cortical centers dedicated to cognition and behavior, insuring our survival. Studies of laboratory animals, as well as MRI and PET imaging studies of humans, have found dramatic activation of the reward centers of our brain with drugs and alcohol.

Mood altering drugs hijack the brain's reward centers, leading to compulsive thoughts and behaviors to acquire the mood-altering substance. Consequently, thoughts and behaviors needed to survive are displaced; all the addict or alcoholic wants to do is more of his or her drug of choice. Neuroscience research using functional MRI and PET imaging has shown that mood-altering drugs directly affect the decision-making centers in our brain, which are intimately related to our reward centers. Under the influence of alcohol or mood-altering substances our judgment is compromised and our ability to make rational choices is limited; we are cognitively impaired.

Drugs and alcohol also affect our hormonal balance through the hypothalamic-pituitary axis. *With exposure to drugs or alcohol the stress hormone, cortisol, is elevated throughout our bodies, which potentiates and perpetuates the addiction and further causes cognitive impairment and damages other organ systems.* Due to the adverse effects on the hypothalamic-pituitary axis and the circulating stress hormone, cortisol, compromised judgment and other cognitive functions may persistent for weeks or months.

Because the mood-altering drug so powerfully stimulates the pleasure centers in our brains, while in active addiction all of our thoughts, attitudes, and behaviors become focused on procuring and using our drug of choice, despite escalating negative consequences. Our behaviors become compulsive. As a dying star collapses into a black hole, the addict's life enters the vortex of addiction and collapses into "self," only to die. Aberrant thinking and behaviors necessary for drinking or using the drug of choice are deplorable to the outside person, but to the addict these are acceptable, as they are required to sustaining the addiction and feeding the screaming, insatiable reward centers. In many cases the changes in thinking and behaviors are subtle and difficult to dissect from normal responses to life's hectic pace, but they tend to progress.

Unless interrupted with an aggressive recovery program, the limbic cravings that feed the aberrant, addictive thinking patterns and behaviors, can last a lifetime—that is, if the addict does not die an early, painful death. It is well-known in the community of alcoholics and addicts that, even after many years of abstinence, exposure to one drink or drug can ignite a cascade of behaviors and attitudes requisite to acquiring the drug or drink. Studies in rats have shown long lasting effects of addiction on the neurotransmitters in the brain: A phenomenon called *"neural sensitization"* of the limbic reward pathways has been described which is responsible for the intense craving and return of addictive use after one drink or drug, even after a long period of abstinence.

The sensitization of limbic reward systems is accompanied by associative learning. Associative learning leads to excessive importance of stimuli associated with drug taking. The sensitization of neural pathways, therefore, transforms ordinary "wanting" into excessive drug "needing," and leads to compulsive drug use. Thus, neural sensitization in the limbic reward centers and related areas can produce addictive behavior (compulsive drug seeking and drug taking), even if the expectation of drug pleasure is diminished, and in the face of strong disincentives, such as the loss of reputation, job, home and family.

Interruption of the death spiral of addiction to alcohol or drugs requires complete abstinence and time to allow brain neurotransmitters and hormones to recover. Levels of neurotransmitters in the addicted brain have been altered and restoring them to normal takes time, usually weeks or months. Although there are several medications that can facilitate early recovery by replacing brain neurotransmitters or blocking receptor sites, residential treatment programs and Twelve-Step programs remain the best-proven methods to achieve sustainable recovery. Residential treatment programs, which usually last thirty to ninety days, are optimal to begin the lifelong process of recovery. The alcoholic or addict brain needs time to heal. Initially, neurotransmitters need to be naturally re-established. Once the brain begins to heal, hormone levels will begin to normalize.

Twelve-Step programs state that by working the Twelve Steps, engaging in meetings, and being of service to others, the obsession to drink or drug is "removed," which is the "miracle" of a "mysterious" process. *I believe recovery is indeed a miracle; however, it is not necessarily a mystery.*

Working the Twelve Steps involves surrendering to a Higher Power and "letting go" of fear, resentment, guilt, self-pity and self-loathing. These emotions are known to be associated with stress physiological states, as exemplified in high autonomic nervous system tone: high blood pressure, elevated respiratory rates, and elevated cortisol (stress hormone) levels. Twelve-Step programs emphasize living along the lines of spiritual principles of honesty, humility, tolerance, patience, acceptance and empathy. Does living a life along these principles reduce stress through re-establishing personal integrity and promoting self-esteem? Can working the Twelve-Steps reduce stress? We will answer these questions in the body of the text.

The 12th Step of Twelve-Step programs promotes altruistic action to promote recovery. Is this rewarding and stress reducing as well? Are empathy and altruism evolutionarily adaptive? Observations of animal societies suggest that empathy and altruism are hard-wired into several mammalian societies. Are humans hard-wired for these virtues as well? I believe the answer is decidedly "yes." This book elaborates on substantial scientific evidence to support this affirmative.

Twelve-Step programs advocate engaging in a relationship with others in fellowship of the specific program. The vast majority of treatment programs use group therapy strategies to promote recovery. Twelve-Step programs—used during initial treatment, and indefinitely thereafter—rely on the *"power of the group"* and relationship with a sponsor for success. Recovering individuals usually attend several Twelve-Step groups per week as an integral component of their recovery program. It is said within circles of recovering addicts and alcoholics that "meeting makers make it," and those who stop attending meetings are substantially more susceptible to relapse into compulsive drug use. This begs the questions: Why is the social experience of the recovery group so integral to recovery? Do empathetic relationships with the fellowship promote happiness and comfort?

Socialization behaviors have been hard-wired into the social brains of numerous animal species throughout the phylogenetic tree, particularly the warm-blooded mammals. Prominent sociobiologists, such as Nobel Laureate E. O. Wilson and others, have long accepted the axiom that socialization behaviors are hard-wired into the brains of many mammalian species, from rodents to canines, primates, and humans, and absolutely are necessary for survival of their species. These species nurse and care for their young and engage in other socialization behaviors promoting survival. What is the neuroscience and physiology behind our instinctive social nature?

Functional magnetic resonance imaging (fMRI) studies of brains in humans and primates during socializing paradigms show activation of the limbic reward centers of the brain, the same centers activated by the drug of choice, during positive, empathetic socialization tasks. Thus, it can be hypothesized that the positive, empathetic socializing experience of the Twelve-Step group makes the addict "feel good," which is why it is essential for recovery. Several empirical studies support this hypothesis and indicate that social reward is processed in the same brain reward centers in the limbic system as non-social reward and drug addiction. Several studies in rodents highlight the importance of limbic ventral striatal (reward center) dopamine for socially motivated behavior, such as maternal care, mating behavior and social attachment.

Data from fMRI studies in humans exhibit ventral striatal (subunit of the limbic system) activations for a variety of rewarding social stimuli, such as beautiful faces, positive emotional expressions, a positive social reputation, and maternal and romantic love. Additionally, recent studies have shown activation of the limbic reward centers in anticipation of positive social feedback. These findings are in line with studies showing neural pathway activations in anticipation of rewarding non-social outcomes such as money, food, or mood-altering drugs. These observations highlight the importance and motivational potential of social stimuli. They also form the basis of our understanding that the "power of the group" may be as strong as the power of the addiction.

Hormonal changes in the recovering addict and alcoholic likely contribute to the healing power of the group. The small peptide hormone, oxytocin—well known to be secreted in lactating mammals and to cause uterine contractions in childbirth—has been implicated in mother-infant bonding. Several lines of study implicate oxytocin in promoting socialization outside of the mother-infant relationship. Oxytocin has been nicknamed the "comfort hormone" or the "tend-and-befriend hormone." Oxytocin has relaxing and calming properties in animals and humans and acts counter to the stress hormone, cortisol. Can oxytocin also contribute to the "power of the group?" We will explore this in the body of this book.

Twelve-Step programs also emphasize the importance of a close connection to a Higher Power, be it the God of our understanding, nature, or the Twelve-Step group itself. These programs also emphasize the role of prayer and meditation and the attainment of a unique and powerful spiritual experience as integral to recovery. Do these spiritual experiences also have neural and hormonal correlates?

A relatively strong consensus has emerged from research studies employing fMRI techniques showing activation of nuclei in the limbic reward system during spiritual experiences in humans. Functional MRI studies of meditating monks and nuns show activity in the frontal and temporal lobes, as well as the limbic system. Brain imaging studies also show that spiritual experiences achieved through intense meditation and prayer decrease activity in the area of the brain that orients our bodies in space, encouraging a blurring of the normal sense of self. This brain activity can stimulate feelings of mystical unity, "oneness," peace, and even the sensed presence of God or other invisible entities.

Do the findings of these studies suggest that our perception of God is fallacious? Certainly not. Temporal lobe and limbic activity may be interpreted within culturally constructed religious assumptions, but should not be confused with the original brain stimuli in the first place. In other words, the spiritual experience activates the brain, but this activation is interpreted in higher cortical centers by cultural conditioning. The spiritual experience may be in the brain, but God is in culture.

Sara Lazar, a researcher at Massachusetts General Hospital and Harvard Medical School, discovered that the more one practices mindfulness meditation, the thicker the brain becomes in the frontal and temporal lobes of the brain, areas responsible for controlling behaviors and emotions. For many years, scientists believed that the brain's plasticity—that is, its ability to create new structures and learn—was limited after childhood. However, current research shows that we can alter the structure of the brain and reap the benefits well into adulthood.

Studies have also shown that meditation reduces the amount of activity in the amygdala, the walnut-sized area in the center of the brain responsible for fear. When the amygdala is relaxed, the parasympathetic nervous system engages to counteract the anxiety response. The heart rate lowers, breathing deepens and slows, and the body stops releasing cortisol and adrenaline into the bloodstream; these stress hormones provide us with quick energy in times of danger but have damaging effects on the body in the long term if they are too prevalent. Studies in meditating Buddhist monks have also revealed lower cortisol levels and decreased stress-reactivity than non-meditators.

By building new neural connections among brain cells in recovery, we rewire the brain, and with each new neural connection, the brain is "re-learning;" it is recovering. It is as if we are adding more RAM to a computer, giving it more functionality. Leading neuroscientists agree that the adult brain is constantly growing new nerve cells and creating new connections leading to the phrase: "Where neurons fire, they can rewire." Neuroscientists agree that one of the benefits of meditation is this process of creating new neural networks for self-observation, optimism, and well-being.

Numerous lines of research have shown that the processes of empathetic social interactions and spiritual practices stimulate the brain's limbic reward centers, normalize hormonal imbalances and, therefore, we can hypothesize that these "natural" rewards replace those of the addictive substance. With empathetic socialization and spiritual practices, stress is reduced, lowering the blood cortisol level, increasing parasympathetic tone and stimulating oxytocin release.

Recovery from addiction requires hard work. It takes time and effort to recapture the reward centers of our brain, as well as their closely associated higher cognitive centers. It takes time for the brain to rewire and hormonal imbalances associated with addiction to normalize. Since 1935,

7

the birth-date of Alcoholics Anonymous, millions of seemingly hopeless alcoholics and addicts have recovered through their efforts in Twelve-Step recovery programs. *It is my hope, armed with the understanding of the neurobiology of addiction and Twelve-Step recovery provided in this book, that more addicts and alcoholics will recover from the painful, humiliating, and seemingly hopeless incarceration of all addictions.*

BOOK I

How Our Brains Are Hijacked by Addictive Drugs and Alcohol

Chapter 1

Addiction: An Insidious, Costly, and Deadly Brain Disease

"I didn't know what to do. I was so depressed, I couldn't think, I couldn't work. All I wanted to do is drink and lay around the house. I didn't enjoy life anymore. I couldn't live with myself. I just wanted to die . . ."

~to paraphrase Robert H., a man I met after an AA meeting many years ago.

I learned later that Robert had tried to kill himself with carbon monoxide from automobile exhaust by running his car in his closed garage. He was discovered by a neighbor who called 911. He had a history of DUI's and had failed court-ordered treatment twice. He was recently fired from his job for alcohol-related issues. Several months prior to our conversation, Robert, while intoxicated, pinned his seven year-old son's leg against a concrete wall with his car while drunk, causing a hairline fracture. Robert was living a nightmare. Robert has the disease of alcoholism. We will follow up with Robert at the close of this chapter.

The Threat of Drug and Alcohol Addiction to Mankind

After millions of years of evolution, we are faced with a substantial challenge to our survival as a human species: drug and alcohol addiction. Every day, millions of people struggle with addiction and millions more watch with feelings of hopelessness, as addiction coldly and systematically destroys the lives of their loved ones. Innocent lives are put at risk by reckless intoxicated addicts with often-horrific consequences. Addiction is a disease, a worldwide epidemic with evolutionary biological, psychological and social ramifications.

Although many organizations have amassed countless survey results and miles of pages of data relating to the effects of drug addiction and alcoholism on society, this information cannot even begin to scratch the surface of the devastation and hopelessness felt by addicts and their families on a daily bases. When a family is struck with addiction, the effects go far beyond numbers and statistics. The emotions of failure, depression, anger, disparity, confusion, and sheer terror that addiction inflicts on its victims and their families are not something any statistic can accurately describe. We can do all we can to educate the public on addiction, but most will tell you that until you go through it, or watch a loved one go through it, there is no way to fully encompass the true effects of drug addiction and alcoholism

Addiction is a disease that affects the brain, constantly giving its host excuses and justification for drug and alcohol abuse. For this reason, addiction is one of the most devastating diseases plaguing our society. Addicts cannot see it until they have lost control, and even then, addiction continues to drive the destructive behavior associated with the disease. Despite trips to the emergency department for alcohol poisoning, drug overdoses, and drug-and alcohol-related accidents and arrests, addicts will continue their abuse. *Addiction has hijacked the brain.*

In many social circles, drug and alcohol abuse are not only acceptable, but also encouraged, giving addiction a huge window of opportunity. There is no way to know when recreational drug and alcohol use will become an addiction, since it is not an immediate onset. The progression of addiction in itself is subtle and grows with each individual's tolerance and continued use of one or multiple substances. Although many who use drugs and alcohol recreationally do not become addicts, millions more do, and a large majority of those people never see it coming. With the socially acceptable nature of alcohol and many drugs in our society, the availability and abuse of these substances have grown to alarming rates.

The more often unsuspecting addicts can get away with drug and alcohol abuse, the more indestructible they feel, thinking they will never be caught or get a DUI. "These things never happen to me," they say, until they happen. Addiction is a very serious problem, and the most disturbing of all facts associated with addiction is that the disease is subtly progressive and more often than not, undetectable by its victims until life is completely out of control, riddled with disparity, financial hardships, and instability. To many addicts, life becomes a deep dark hole. With such devastating consequences, it would seem logical not to take the risk for addiction in the first place. However, despite the vast amounts of information available about addiction and the dangers therein, our society remains disturbingly more focused on the temporary enjoyment of mood-altering drugs and alcohol rather than the permanently devastating depression and damage caused by drug and alcohol addiction.

The National Institute on Drug Addiction (NIDA, 2008) estimates that 22 million Americans suffered from drug and alcohol addiction, as determined from treatment center admissions data only. The National Institute on Alcohol Abuse and Alcoholism (NIAAA) informs us that alcoholism kills approximately 100,000 Americans every year, and is the third leading preventable cause of death in the United States next to cancer and heart disease.

Globally, the use of addictive mood-altering drugs has increased year after year. On average, drug popularity differs from nation to nation. The United Nations Office on Drugs and Crime identified major problem drugs by analyzing treatment demand by each continent (UNDOC, 2004). From 1998 to 2003, Asia, Europe, and Australia showed major problems with opiate addiction, South America was affected predominantly by cocaine addiction, and Africans were treated most often for cannabis addiction. In North America, drug addiction was distributed relatively evenly among opiates, cannabis, cocaine, amphetamines, and other narcotics. The report showed, however, that all types of drugs are consumed throughout each continent. Interpol reported that over 4,000 tons of cannabis were seized in 1999, up 20 percent from 1998, with the largest seizures made in Southern Africa, the United States, Mexico, and Western Europe (Saah, 2005). Almost 150 tons of cocaine are purchased each year throughout Europe, and in 1999 opium production reached an estimated 6,600 tons, the dramatic increase most likely due to robust poppy crops throughout Southwest Asia.

In 2008, 51.6 percent of Americans age 12 and older had used alcohol at least once in the 30 days prior to being surveyed; 23.3 percent had binged (5+ drinks within 2 hours); and 23.3 percent drank heavily (5+ drinks on 5+ occasions). In the 12 to 17 age range, 14.6 percent had consumed at least one drink in the 30 days prior to being surveyed; 8.8 percent had binged; and 2.0 percent drank heavily (NIDA, 2008).

The Bureau of Justice reports an estimated 1,654,000 drug related arrests for adults 18 years and up in 2005, up over 60 percent from 1,008,300 in 1990 (NIDA, 2005). According to the National Highway Traffic Safety Administration (NHTSA), there were 17,941 alcohol related traffic fatalities in 2006, a 4 percent increase from 2005 (NHTSA, 2007). These numbers have been on a steady increase since 1970, and will likely continue with the wide availability of both legal and illegal drugs. The World Health Organization cited almost 200,000 drug-induced deaths alone in the year 2000 (UNIO, 2005).

According to NHTSA statistics, drunk driving results in an injury every minute and one death every 32 minutes. In the United States, about 40 percent of traffic-related casualties are linked to alcohol use. Crime rates go up because of addiction related incidents. In 1992, over 25 percent of violent crimes and property crimes were attributed to drug and alcohol abuse. Substance abuse impairs the individual's productivity. It can affect his ability to maintain a full-time job. In cases where addicts are even able to maintain employment, the people around them are placed at risk. Thirty-four percent of social welfare cases in the country were caused by substance abuse.

The economic cost of drug, alcohol, and tobacco abuse in the United States is nearly $500 billion, and impacts 100 million people's lives, either directly or indirectly (NIDA, 2008). This is more than the total costs associated with diabetes and cancer combined. The estimated economic impact of alcohol-related crashes in the United States is $15.7 million. Alcohol-involved crashes resulted in 16,792 fatalities, 513,000 nonfatal injuries, and $50.9 billion in economic costs in 2000, accounting for 22 percent of all crash costs. Drugs, often in combination with alcohol, are used by approximately 10 to 22 percent of drivers involved in crashes. Drugged driving causes $33 billion in damages every year. Children with prenatal cocaine exposure are 1.5 times more likely than non-exposed children to need special education services in school. Special-education costs for this population are estimated at $23 million per year.

According to studies by NIDA and NIAAA, the younger a person first uses drugs or alcohol, the greater the likelihood that they will become dependent on and/or addicted to drugs and alcohol as an adult (NIDA, 2008). Youth who first smoke marijuana under the age of 14 are more than five times as likely to abuse drugs in adulthood. Forty-five percent of youth who began drinking before age 15 were classified as dependent later in life whereas of youth who began drinking between the ages of 17 and 21, 24.5 percent were classified as dependent, and of youth who began drinking at age 21 or 22, 10 percent were classified as dependent. Understandably, the NIDA and NIAAA reports plead for prevention.

The Disease Model of Addiction ⟶ *Like a virus, its chronic & progressive*

There are large volumes of scientific literature showing that addictive drugs target the brain, specifically its reward pathways (Berridge, 1998; Robinson, 1993). The reward pathways evolved to promote activities that are essential to the survival of the human race, as well as other animals lower on the phylogenetic tree, such as successful reproduction and procurement of adequate nutrition. This reinforcement pathway, which is composed of both central nervous system structures and endogenous neurotransmitters communicating between these structures, is located in the middle/center of the brain called the limbic system.

One may compare the mechanism of drug addiction with that of viruses. Viruses and drugs of abuse are both pathogenic agents for humans. Viruses enter an animal's cells and use the host cell's core subunits for survival—DNA and RNA—to synthesize more viruses, thus promoting their own survival. As the new viruses infect more and more cells, the host suffers symptoms or may perish. Illicit drugs affect their host in a similar fashion. Just as viruses hijack a cell's RNA and DNA, drugs of abuse hijack the brain's core reward pathway to promote continued use. Just as the cell's survival is dependent on its core DNA and RNA, so is the survival of the organism dependent on an intact brain reward pathway. By hijacking the brain's reward pathways, drugs of abuse—through changes in emotions, cognitive function, and behaviors—all too frequently lead to severely negative consequences for the host/user, including death.

The disease model of addiction also proposes that addiction is a chronic, progressive disease, like the slow-acting virus of HIV infection, or other chronic progressive diseases such as diabetes, and cardiovascular disease. This popular model of addiction is credited to E.M. Jellinek (1960) who presented a comprehensive disease model of alcoholism in 1960. Addiction is considered to fit the definition of a medical ailment, involving an abnormality of structure in, or function of, the brain that results in behavioral impairment. At the heart of this model or theory is that addiction is characterized by a person's inability to control his or her use of alcohol or drugs, and that person develops an uncontrollable craving or compulsion to drink alcohol or take drugs.

The loss of control can be manifested during either a short or long time span. A person may begin what he believes will be a short drinking session, but after one or two drinks he finds it impossible to stop drinking. This phenomenon is described as the *"phenomenon of craving."* "Craving" was defined by E.M. Jellinek, a key player in the development of the disease model, as an *"urgent and overpowering desire."* It can be viewed as a feeling that compels the person to do whatever it takes to obtain the object of the addiction, even when there are potential harmful consequences. The disease model assumes that the impaired control and craving are irreversible. Addiction cannot be cured; it can only be arrested. Like other diseases, there is a natural progression characterized by deterioration of the health of the host, until the host dies.

What Is a Disease?

To discuss intelligently the issue of whether or not addiction is a disease, we must first define the term *"disease."* According to the twenty-eighth Edition of the Stedman's Medical Dictionary, the definition of *"disease"* is:

> *"A morbus, an illness, and a sickness that causes an interruption, cessation, or disorder of bodily functions, systems, or organs. A disease is an entity characterized by at least two of these criteria:*
> *(1) A recognized etiologic agent (or agents): i.e., the causes*
> *(2) Consistent anatomical alterations of known body systems*
> *(3) An identifiable group of signs and symptoms"*

To determine if drug and alcohol addiction is a disease, we must see if it meets these three criteria (Gorski, 2003).

What Are the Causes of Addiction and Alcoholism?

The etiology of alcoholism and drug addiction is best understood as a complex interaction between genetic and environmental factors (Gorski, 2003). The World Health Organization (WHO) provides a model for understanding the role of environmental factors in the etiology of the disease of addiction. According to this model, host biological and genetic factors interact with environmental factors to produce disease. *The WHO model recognizes three basic elements of the disease of addiction: (1) a susceptible host, (2) a toxic agent, and (3) a permissive environment (WHO, 2007).* First, it is evident that different people have different susceptibility to addiction once they ingest alcohol and/or drugs. There is substantial evidence that there is a genetic predisposition to alcohol and/or drug addiction. Other individuals have psychological issues that predispose them to substance abuse (Everitt, 2001). Second, in addiction the toxic agent is alcohol and/or drugs. The exposure to alcohol or drugs is a necessary catalyst for the development of the disease in a susceptible host. And third, the social environment will increase or decrease the likelihood of exposure to and the abuse of the toxic agent (alcohol and/or drugs). The more a society reinforces the use of drugs and alcohol as necessary or desirable the greater the likelihood that more members of the culture will be exposed to the toxic agent (Ellickson, 2003).

GENETICS AND ENVIRONMENT

Genetic Predisposition

The heritability of risk for alcohol dependence is similar to type 2 diabetes. The heritability risk has been estimated by studies of the adopted-away offspring of affected and unaffected parents as 39 percent (Cloninger, 1981), and 60 percent by twin studies (Heath, 1997; NIAAA, 1992). Similar rates of heritability for other types of drug addiction have been indicated by other studies (Kendler, 1994, Bierut, 1998). We know that if you have one parent with alcoholism, the chance of an offspring having it is 40 percent. An estimated 20 to 25 percent of sons and brothers of alcoholics become alcoholics, as stated from the UCSF Family Alcoholism Study, while 5 percent of daughters and sisters of alcoholics become alcoholics (UCSF Family Alcoholism Study, 2002). Cotton (1979), in her classic review of family studies, concluded that alcoholics were six times more likely than non-alcoholics to report a positive family history of alcoholism. The general population however has only about a 10 percent risk of having addiction.

According to twin studies, if you have an identical twin who is an alcoholic, then you have about a 60 percent chance of also having alcoholism (Kendler, 1994; Prescott, 1999). However, if alcoholism were purely genetic, then there would be a 100 percent chance the other twin certainly would have addiction as well. In reality, though, it is only 60 percent because this disease, while it has a genetic component, is not 100 percent genetic. *The expression of substance abuse is dependent on genetic liability as well as environmental influences.*

Many studies have been conducted looking for specific chromosomes (genes) for alcoholism. Two studies by the Collaborative Study on the Genetics of Alcoholism (COGA) of 987 individuals from 105 families containing at least three first-degree relatives with alcohol dependence suggest that there is a strong link between chromosomes 1 and 7 and susceptibility to alcohol dependence, and weak evidence for linkage to chromosome 2 (Edinberg, 2002). Another suspect of genes that was also looked at is a marker known as the dopamine D2 receptor, found by Blum and co-workers to exist more often in alcoholics than non-alcoholics (Blum, 1990).

Population and family studies, such as those cited above, attempt to establish the presence of a broad genetic influence on alcoholism. To investigate specific genes, researchers have employed genetic marker studies. If specific human genes are related to alcoholism, then genes laying close to them on the same chromosome, and the traits they determine, may be inherited at the same time that the risk of alcoholism is inherited. Genetic markers are proteins, partial genes, or DNA sequences that are transmitted from one generation and are close enough on the same chromosome that they do not become separated at gametogenesis (gene duplication) (Palmer, 1991).

The serotonergic neurotransmitter system has been studied as a risk factor for addictive behavior. In particular, the 5-HT serotonin transporter gene (5-HTT) and the 5-HT1B receptor gene have been considered as candidate genes. A functional polymorphism in the 5-HTT promoter was shown to affect 5-HT uptake in lymphoblastic cells (Edenberg, 1998*b*). A study of 319 Germans showed that the frequency of the "short" allele of this gene in the severely affected alcoholics was significantly higher than that in the controls (Sander, 1997). Opioid neurotransmission has also been studied in connection with alcoholism. One study found an association of a polymorphic CAn repeat in the gene OPRM1 locus, which encodes the m-opioid receptor, with alcohol dependence in 320 Caucasian and 108 African American substance-dependent subjects. The

STUDIES W/ MICE/RATS

CAn repeat was significantly more prevalent in the substance-dependent subjects than in the control population (Kranzler, 1998).

The genetic predisposition to alcohol and drug addiction is easy to study in rat populations. Scientists have bred lines of rats that manifest specific and separate alcohol-related traits or phenotypes, such as sensitivity to alcohol's intoxicating and sedative effects, the development of tolerance, the susceptibility to withdrawal symptoms, and alcohol–related organ damage (Liang, 2003, 2010). When a population of randomly selected rats is offered food, water, and alcohol, generally about 10 percent of the rats will prefer the alcohol to the food or water. If you take the 10 percent that prefer the alcohol and breed them, you get a population of 100 percent alcoholic-only-preferring strain of mice. In addition, these alcoholic rats have been observed to behave alcoholically (Liang, 2003, 2010; Bell, 2009). They would drink and, drink and then they would pass out. Often they would fight over the alcohol. Many drank themselves to death. Similar strains of rats have been bred to prefer cocaine to food and water (Crabbe, 1999).

Research in rats and other animals has shown that genes for the brain's reward center pathway receptors may contribute to substance abuse (Vanyukov, 2000). When studied in animals, dopamine D2 receptor has been associated with brain functions relating to reward, reinforcement, and motivation and, therefore, is suspected to increase an individual's risk of alcoholism and other addictions. The genetic liability may be a result of a genetic polymorphism within the D2 dopamine receptor gene (A.sub.1 allele) (Blum, 1990). This particular receptor gene polymorphism correlates with alcohol and substance addiction as well as obsessive-compulsive disorders. The D4 dopamine receptor has documented polymorphisms and correlates with substance addiction. It is believed to be involved in reducing sensitivity to methamphetamines, alcohol, and cocaine. In Israeli and Arab heroin-dependent populations, there was data collected displaying a DRD4 gene polymorphism in chromosome 3 consisting of seven-repeat alleles not present in non-addicted control groups (Phillips, 1991). This was also observed in a study of heroin-addicted Han Chinese. In a study done with Native American alcoholics, a linkage on chromosome 11 near the DRD4 gene was documented (Cravchik, 2000).

The genetic marker that has been suggested to be indicative of a genetic predisposition to alcoholism is also related to the dopaminergic system. It is the A1 allele of the gene for the dopamine D2 receptor. The original 1990 study by Blum, et al. was a post-mortem of thirty-five alcoholics and thirty-five non-alcoholics who found the A1 allele to be present in 69 percent of the alcoholics as opposed to 20 percent of the non-alcoholics. The alcoholics had repeatedly failed treatment, and many of the deaths were alcohol-related. Subsequent studies have generally upheld the initial results, though some have refuted them. One hypothesis is that the A1 allele codes for a lower density of D2 receptors than the more common A2 allele, resulting in an inherited deficit in brain reward mechanisms (Uhl, 1998).

Rates of alcohol, marijuana, and cocaine dependence and habitual smoking were increased in siblings of alcohol-dependent individuals compared with siblings of controls. For siblings of alcohol-dependent individuals, 49.3 to 50.1 percent of brothers and 22.4 to 25.0 percent of sisters were alcohol dependent (lifetime diagnosis), but this elevated risk was not further increased by comorbid substance dependence in individuals (Bierut, 1998). Siblings of marijuana-dependent individuals had an elevated risk of developing marijuana dependence (relative risk, 1.78) and siblings of cocaine-dependent individuals had an elevated risk of developing cocaine dependence (relative risk, 1.71). There was a similar finding for habitual smoking (relative risk, 1.77) in siblings of habitual-smoking individuals). Abuse of cocaine, sedatives, opiates, hallucinogens, and amphetamines, for example, was found to be ten times higher in alcoholics than in non-alcoholics in the Epidemiological Catchment Area (ECA) survey (NCAAD, 2002). However, tentative evidence from other studies suggests caution in assuming that possible genetic bases for predisposition to alcoholism are identical to genetic bases for predisposition to substance abuse. Identification of the specific genetic determinants shared by substance-addicted individuals in general, and those that might be specific to each group of agents, remains an area of current research.

Psychological and Social Factors in the Etiology of Addiction

The etiology of drug addiction has been described as three-fold: biological, psychological, and social. Although humans may be biologically and psychologically predisposed to drug use and addiction, they may often be driven toward that state by social and cultural influences. To what extent environmental stimuli affect a person's vulnerability to addiction is unknown and may vary. However, we cannot ignore the great impact of environmental stimuli in the progression toward addiction. It has been found that certain environmental variables lead to higher vulnerability (Kendler, 2003; Kalivas, 2005). Family dysfunction and disruption, low social-class rearing, poor parental monitoring, and rampant social drug-use exposure may greatly contribute to an individual's movement from substance abuse predisposition to addiction. The widespread availability of drugs in certain areas also may affect susceptibility (SAMHSA, 2004). This is exceptionally notable in low socioeconomic areas in which overcrowding and poverty have been associated statistically with increased substance abuse. In addition, repeated exposure to successful high-status role models who use substances—whether these role models are figures in the media, peers, or older siblings—is likely to influence children and adolescents. Similarly, the perception that smoking, drinking, or drug use is standard practice among peers also serves to promote substance abuse.

Social development and adjustment factors also play a role in drug abuse and addiction. An assumption of the developmental perspective, as mentioned by Jainchill (2000), is that the course of one's life is a process in which life circumstances change, milestones are met or missed, and new social roles are created, while old ones are abandoned. There are well-known and widely accepted norms about when certain developmental events should happen in a person's life. Studies of the social factors involved in drug use have mostly focused on either adolescence or young adulthood, but surprisingly a significant amount of cocaine users may not initiate use until middle adulthood. The majority of people enter into adult social roles on schedule. However, some people enter these roles earlier or later than their same-age peers do. The developmental perspective predicts that this will lead to less-than-satisfactory adjustment, incumbent stress, and possibly self-medication with drugs and alcohol (Neurgarten, 1973; Vlahov, 2002; Khantzian, 1985).

There is also convincing evidence that psychological and social factors can increase the risk of future alcohol abuse and alcoholism (NHSDA, 2004). There is an interaction among personality style, lifestyle, culture, and social system. When these psychosocial variables encourage the following behaviors related to alcohol and drug use, the prevalence of addiction increases. Psychosocial factors that promote drug use and increase the risk for addiction are those that: (1) promote the use of alcohol and drugs as safe, normal, and low-risk behaviors, (2) support frequent use, (3) support heavy use, (4) promote intoxication as normal, and (5) view intoxication as a reason to exempt individuals from personal responsibility.

Stress as a Predominant Psychological Etiology

Certain individuals begin to abuse drugs and alcohol in an attempt to self-medicate their seemingly intolerable states of mind—that is, they self-medicate (Khantzian, 1985). The self-medication theory has a long history. In 1884, Sigmund Freud first raised this concept in noting the anti-depressant properties of cocaine. Stress has long been recognized as a major contributor for drug cravings and relapses. In line with the self-medication theory, a person's use of a particular drug of choice is not an accident, but rather it is chosen for its pharmacological effect in relieving stressful symptoms or unwanted feelings. Research has shown that people who survive disasters are prone to stress related disorders, such as posttraumatic stress disorder (PTSD) and depression. People who experience major trauma in their life may self-medicate with drugs or alcohol to relieve the symptoms of PTSD and depression (Dansky, 1994). These individuals are at greater risk for developing addiction than the general population. The research on the stress and addiction is extensive; therefore, I have dedicated an entire chapter for its elaboration (Chapter 5).

Comorbidity of Psychiatric Illness and Substance Abuse

Data from a number of sources indicate Substance-use disorders and some psychiatric disorders occur concurrently in many individuals. Patients with comorbid conditions are given the designation: "dual diagnosis." Two epidemiological surveys have examined the prevalence of psychiatric and substance use disorders in community samples: the National Institute of Mental Health Epidemiologic Catchment Area (ECA) study (Regier, 1990) conducted in the early 1980s, and the National Co-morbidity Study (NCS) conducted in 1991 (Kessler, 1994) Data from the ECA study estimates that 45 percent of individuals with an alcohol use disorder and 72 percent of individuals with a drug use disorder had at least one co-occurring psychiatric disorder (Kessler, 1994). In the NCS, approximately 78 percent of alcohol-dependent men and 86 percent of alcohol-dependent women met lifetime criteria for another psychiatric disorder, including drug dependence (Kessler, 1994, 1997). Depression and anxiety most commonly occur in the drug addict or alcoholic.

What "Alterations in Known Body Systems" Are Caused by Addiction?

Substances of abuse target the brain reward pathway, which is made of neurons that release chemicals when they are stimulated. This release leads to subjective feelings of well-being (Lowinson, 1997, Koob, 1997). This brain reward system evolved to sub-serve activities essential to species survival, such as sexual activity and feeding behaviors. Activities that activate this pathway become associated with "feeling good." For example, sexual intercourse causes the release of chemicals activating this pathway, and the result is a feeling of well-being. Thus, the reward pathway serves to promote survival of the species by rewarding behaviors necessary for continued survival (seeking food, reproduction, shelter, drink, etc).

Drugs of abuse stimulate this "brain reward" pathway in a similar fashion, and this is why substance users experience feelings of pleasure, or "high," when they use them (Bardo, 1998, Berridge, 1998). When drugs of abuse are repeatedly used, they may "hijack" the brain reward system, driving compulsory drug use to the exclusion of other adaptive activities. Thus, addiction can be partially explained by the action of drugs of abuse on this common reward pathway, in which drug use stimulates further use and drug-seeking behavior (Joseph, 1996).

Studies have shown that drugs of abuse also affect the endocrine (hormone) system. The neurotransmitters of our brain and the hormones of our endocrine system control our perceptions, cognition, and expressions. They regulate our physical and mental homeostatic processes and our natural rhythm cycles, such as activity and rest, eating and digestion, exploration and survival, as well as all other human states or moods. The constant temperature of our bodies is a testament to the magnificent architecture and precise interaction of our body's nervous and endocrine systems. The mutual needs of these biological partners define our motivational drive and are expressed in our emotional responses.

The effect of alcohol on the body deserves separate mention, because there is a definite profile of alcohol-related damage to body systems and organs that usually does not occur in people who do not have alcoholism.

The major organ system that is affected is the brain. There is clear evidence from neuropsychological studies that alcoholics have cognitive impairments related to the organic damage caused by chronic alcohol poisoning to the brain (Muller, 1985). The American Psychiatric Association's *Diagnostic and Statistical Manual of Mental Disorders* (DSM-IV) clearly identifies and differentiates "substance-related organic mental disorders" and describes their direct correlation to alcoholism. Many other organ systems are also affected. The liver, pancreas, heart, endocrine systems, among others, are all affected. In many cases, alcoholism is fatal, because if the alcoholic continues to drink heavily and regularly, multiple organ systems will fail (Lowinson, 1997).

What Are the "Signs and Symptoms" of Addiction?

The disease of addiction is marked by predictable signs and symptoms. The definite progression of symptoms is, in part, related to a pathologically altered brain reward mechanism. The DSM-IV (1994) places a heavy weight upon the *pattern of compulsive use* as the primary factor distinguishing between abuse and dependence. The DSM-IV has categorized three stages of addiction: preoccupation and anticipation, binge and intoxication, and withdrawal and negative affect (mood). These stages are characterized, respectively, everywhere by constant cravings and preoccupation with obtaining the substance; using more of the substance than necessary to experience the intoxicating effects; and experiencing tolerance, withdrawal symptoms, and decreased motivation for normal life activities. According to the DSM-IV, the pattern of compulsive use is marked by the following signs and symptoms:

1. *Craving: A strong desire to use the substance.*
2. *Tolerance and loss of control over use: The tendency to use larger quantities of the substance than intended and to use the substance for longer periods of time than intended.*
3. *Inability to abstain: The persistent desire to cut down or control accompanied by the failure to be able to so in spite of past attempts.*
4. *Addiction Centered Lifestyle: The increased amount of time spent in seeking and using alcohol and other drugs resulting in the centering of major life activities around alcohol and drug use.*

5. *Addictive Lifestyle Losses: The tendency to give up or reduce the frequency of involvement in important life activities to accommodate the increased amount of time spent in drug seeking and using.*

6. *Continued Use In Spite of Negative Consequences: The tendency to continue to use alcohol and drugs in spite of negative consequences.*

Therefore, according to the American Psychiatric Association, it is appropriate to describe people with severe alcohol or drug problems that meet the DSM-IV criteria of substance dependence as having a disease. In these cases, there is clear evidence of a syndrome, with clearly identifiable patterns of signs and symptoms, and a disorder, with clear evidence that those signs and symptoms have created both functional and structural impairment. According to the DSM-IV, the diagnosis of substance (drug) dependence requires at least three of the above symptoms.

Several addictionologists have further elaborated on the DSM-IV's symptom list. Prominent addictionologist Terence Gorski elaborated on signs and symptoms referred to in the DSM-IV and described a progression of pathological thoughts and behaviors related to progressive pathological alteration of the brain's reward system. The following are paraphrased from his web site (Gorski, 2003):

1. *Chronic Low Grade Agitated Depression: The addicted individual experiences a chronic state of low-grade agitated depression due to abnormally low release of brain reward chemicals. This state is dysphoric and generates an urge to find something—anything— that will relieve this state.*

2. *Biological Reinforcement: The addicted person takes his drug of choice, which activates the release of brain reward chemicals. This results in an intense feeling of euphoria and personal well-being. Negative feelings are mitigated. Drug use is reinforced.*

3. *Obsession, Compulsion, and Craving: The biological reinforcement stimulates the brain's limbic system to develop an emotional urge to repeat the experience. This emotional urge can be described as a "primitive tissue hunger" or craving for the drug.*

3. *Tolerance: The person is able to use large amounts of the drug of choice without becoming intoxicated or impaired. As a result he can use heavily without apparent adverse consequences.*

4. *Hangover Resistance: The person experiences minimal sickness on the morning after using alcohol and drugs. This rapid recovery allows the person to resume use rapidly and to use the drug of choice frequently.*

5. *Addictive Beliefs: As a result of the experiences created by the biological reinforcement, craving, high tolerance, and hangover resistance, the individual comes to believe that the drug of choice is good for him and will magically fix him or make him better. He violates his own moral code to use his drug of choice.*

6. *Addictive Lifestyle: The addicted individual attracts, and is attracted to, other individuals who share strong positive attitudes toward the use of alcohol and other drugs. They become immersed in an addiction-centered subculture.*

7. *Addictive Lifestyle Losses: The person distances himself from people who support sobriety and surrounds himself with people who support alcohol and drug use. He avoids normal responsibilities. Avoiding responsibilities is considered normal in the drug subculture.*

8. *A Pattern of Heavy and Regular Use: The biological reinforcement has motivated the person to build a belief system and lifestyle that supports heavy and regular use. The person is now in a state where hy uses larger amounts with greater frequency despite physical, psychological and social degeneration.*

9. *Progressive Neurological and Neuropsychological Impairments: The progressive damage of alcohol and drugs to the brain creates growing problems with judgment and impulse control. As a result, behavior begins to spiral out of control. The cognitive capacities needed to think abstractly about the problem have also been impaired and the person is locked into a pattern marked by denial and impaired reasoning.*

10. *Denial: The addict is unable to recognize the pattern of problems related to the use of alcohol and drugs when problems are experienced and confronted.*

11. *Degeneration: The addict begins to experience physical, psychological and social deterioration. Unless the person develops an unexpected insight, the progressive problems are likely to continue until confronted by or intervened by others.*

12. *Inability to Abstain: The person attempts to abstain but is plagued by acute withdrawal and the longer-term withdrawal symptoms associated with chronic brain toxicity. In addiction, the initial low-grade agitated depression and symptoms of anhedonia are magnified. When*

coupled with cognitive impairment, addictive belief systems and the deeply ingrained pattern of obsession, compulsion, and craving, the addict finds himself unable to maintain abstinence.

13. *Vulnerability to relapse: An addict, after a sustained period of abstinence, is prone to relapse in to active using, its associated behaviors and attitudes, and personal and social consequences.*

The disease of addiction involves the progression of acute drug use to the development of drug-seeking behavior, the vulnerability to relapse, and the decreased, slowed ability to respond to naturally rewarding stimuli. It is apparent that a motivation or physiological drive stronger than our conscious concerns is at work fueling addictive behaviors. Addiction means giving up conscious control. It is impulsive, unconscious behavior. As it is said in Alcoholics (or Narcotics) Anonymous, "Addicts are people who have lost all control of their lives," as well as their substance use and abuse. These people have tried many different times to stop using these substances—for their own personal, financial, or social reasons—and yet they could not. They were able to stop for short periods, or curb use for longer periods, but true abstinence over an extended period is somewhat rare among true addicts. Also, addiction is a progressive, chronic disease. Unless the addictive cycle is interrupted through intervention, treatment, and a sound recovery program, the addicted individual will generally sacrifice all that is important in life for the sake of using or drinking and, sadly, many die from secondary effects of the addictive substance (e.g., overdose, organ failure), accidents or suicides.

Institutional Adoption of the Disease Model of Addiction

The belief that alcohol and drug addiction is a disease is promoted by numerous organizations, including the World Health Organization (WHO), the American Medical Association (AMA), and the American Psychiatric Association (APA). The U.S. Congress formally acknowledged that alcoholism was a disease with the passage of the Hughes Act in 1970. The National Institute on Alcohol Abuse and Alcoholism (NIAAA) was created to promote research on the nature of this disease. A major thrust of NIAAA has been on the biomedical aspects of this disease and much progress has been made in understanding its etiology, symptoms, and treatment.

The term "addiction" has been defined and re-defined over the years. In 1957 the World Health Organization (WHO) Expert Committee on Addiction-Producing Drugs defined addiction as: *". . . a state of periodic or chronic intoxication produced by the repeated consumption of a drug (natural or synthetic). Its characteristics include: (i) an overpowering desire or need (compulsion) to continue taking the drug and to obtain it by any means; (ii) a tendency to increase the dose; (iii) a psychic (psychological) and generally a physical dependence on the effects of the drug; and (iv) detrimental effects on the individual and on society . . ."* (WHO, 1957)

The WHO distinguishes drug addiction from habituation by stating: *"Drug habituation (habit) is a condition resulting from the repeated consumption of a drug. Its characteristics include (i) a desire (but not a compulsion) to continue taking the drug for the sense of improved well-being which it engenders; (ii) little or no tendency to increase the dose; (iii) some degree of psychic dependence on the effect of the drug, but absence of physical dependence and hence of an abstinence syndrome (withdrawal), and (iv) detrimental effects, if any, primarily on the individual."*

In 1964, the WHO committee further redefined these terms, and suggested using the generic term *"drug dependence."* In their proceedings they state: *"The definition of addiction gained some acceptance, but confusion in the use of the terms addiction and habituation and misuse of the former continued. Further, the list of drugs abused increased in number and diversity. These difficulties have become increasingly apparent and various attempts have been made to find a term that could be applied to drug abuse generally. The component in common appears to be dependence, whether psychic or physical or both. Hence, use of the term "drug dependence," with a modifying phase linking it to a particular drug type in order to differentiate one class of drugs from another, had been given most careful consideration. The Expert Committee recommends substitution of the term "drug dependence" for the terms "drug addiction" and "drug habituation."* (WHO, 1964)

In 2004, the World Health Organization's International Statistical Classification of Diseases and Related Health Problems (ICD) published a detailed report on alcohol and other psychoactive substances titled "Neuroscience of psychoactive substance use and dependence" (WHO, 2004). It stated that this was the *"first attempt by WHO to provide a comprehensive overview of the biological factors related to substance use and dependence by summarizing the vast amount of knowledge gained in the last 20-30 years. The report highlights the current state of knowledge of the mechanisms of action of different types of psychoactive substances, and explains how the use of these substances can lead to the development of dependence syndrome."* The report further states that *"dependence has not previously been recognized as a disorder of the brain, in the same way that psychiatric and mental illnesses were not previously viewed as being a result of a disorder of the brain. However, with recent advances in neuroscience, it is clear that dependence is as much a disorder of the brain as any other neurological or psychiatric illness."*

The American Academy of Pain Medicine, the American Pain Society, and the American Society of Addiction Medicine jointly issued "Definitions Related to the Use of Opioids for the Treatment of Pain" in 2001 which provided the following definition: *"Addiction is a primary, chronic, neurobiological disease, with genetic, psychosocial, and environmental factors influencing its development and manifestations. It is characterized by behaviors that include one or more of the following: impaired control over drug use, compulsive use, continued use despite harm, and craving . . . . Physical dependence is a state of adaptation that is manifested by a drug class specific withdrawal syndrome that can be produced by abrupt cessation, rapid dose reduction, decreasing blood level of the drug, and/or administration of an antagonist . . . . Tolerance is the body's physical adaptation to a drug: greater amounts of the drug are required over time to achieve the initial effect as the body "gets used to" and adapts to the intake."* (ASAM, 2001)

Although the 1957 and 1964 definitions of addiction, dependence and abuse persist to the present day in medical literature, it should be noted that at this time (2011) the fourth edition of the DSM-IV uses the term *"substance dependence"* instead of *"addiction."* In the modern medical profession, the two most used diagnostic tools in the world—the American Psychiatric Association's *Diagnostic and Statistical Manual of Mental Disorders* (DSM-IV) and the World Health Organization's *International Statistical Classification of Diseases and Related Health Problems*—no longer recognize *"drug abuse"* as a current medical diagnosis. Instead, the DSM-IV has adopted *"substance dependence"* as a blanket term to include drug abuse and other things. The WHO recognizes the terminology: *"drug dependence syndrome."*

Physical dependence on, abuse of, and withdrawal from drugs and other miscellaneous substances are outlined in the DSM-IV. The DSM-IV section on substance dependence begins with the following: *"Substance dependence: When an individual persists in use of alcohol or other drugs despite problems related to use of the substance, substance dependence may be diagnosed. Compulsive and repetitive use may result in tolerance to the effect of the drug and withdrawal symptoms when use is reduced or stopped. These, along with Substance Abuse are considered Substance Use Disorders . . ."*

Addictive Potential of Drugs and Alcohol

Drugs known to cause addiction include illegal drugs as well as prescription or over-the-counter drugs, according to the definition by the American Society of Addiction Medicine. Addictive drugs may be classified as follows:

- *Stimulants:*

  Amphetamine and methamphetamine
  Cocaine
  Nicotine

- *Sedatives and hypnotics:*

  Alcohol
  Barbiturates
  Benzodiazepines, particularly flunitrazepam, triazolam,
      temazepam, and nimetazepam
  Methaqualone and the related quinazolinone
      sedative-hypnotics

- *Opiate and opioid analgesics:*

  Morphine and codeine, the two naturally occurring opiate
      analgesics
  Semi-synthetic opiates, such as heroin (diacetylmorphine),
      oxycodone, buprenorphine, and hydromorphone
  Fully synthetic opioids, such as fentanyl, meperidine/pethidine,
      and methadone

- *Cannabis:*

  Marijuana, Hashish, THC resin

- *Hallucinogens:*

LSD, mescaline, PCP

- *Designer drugs:*

Designer drugs are manufactured (designed) from other drugs. The three main drugs that serve as the basis for 'designer drugs' are PCP, fentanyl, and amphetamine/methamphetamine. Once 'changed,' they become known by a variety of street names—for example, XTC, Ecstasy, Adam, Lover's Speed, Special K, Fantasy and Nature's Quaalude. They are sold as tablets or capsules to produce feelings of stimulation and euphoria, a sense of well-being, and various sensory distortions. Higher doses can lead to paranoia, hallucinations, violent or otherwise irrational behavior, and fatal overdoses.

The addictive potential of a drug varies from substance to substance, and from individual to individual. Dose, frequency, pharmacokinetics of a particular substance, route of administration, and time are critical factors for developing a drug addiction. An article in *The Lancet* compared the harm and addiction of twenty drugs, using a scale from 0 to 3 for physical addiction, psychological addiction, and pleasure to create a mean score for addiction. Selected results can be seen in the chart below (from Nutt, 2007):

Drug	Mean	Pleasure	Psychological Dependence	Physical Dependence
Heroin	3.00	3.0	3.0	3.0
Cocaine	2.37	3.0	2.8	1.3
Alcohol	2.23	2.3	2.6	1.8
Tobacco	2.23	2.3	2.6	1.8
Barbiturates	2.01	2.0	2.2	1.8
Benzodiazepines	1.83	1.7	2.1	1.8
Amphetamine	1.67	2.0	1.9	1.1
Cannabis	1.47	1.9	1.7	0.8
LSD	1.23	2.2	1.1	0.3
Ecstasy	1.13	1.5	1.2	0.7

Having a Disease is NOT an Excuse

At this point, I must emphasize my personal position as a recovering alcoholic: The fact that drug and alcohol addiction is a recognized disease does not excuse the irresponsible behaviors of an addict or alcoholic. The substantial difference between the disease of addiction and other chronic diseases, like diabetes, is the irresponsible behaviors of the addict and alcoholic and their toll on innocent bystanders and society as a whole. My heart aches knowing the hardships I placed on my family and my employer while I struggled in my addiction to alcohol. I am uncomfortable sitting in an Alcoholics Anonymous room next to someone who caused bodily injury or death to another as a consequence of his active, untreated disease. As stated previously, our entire society pays the enormous cost of addiction and alcoholism.

As this book will address, the disease of addiction manifests itself as a loss of decision-making skills and other executive functions. The active addict and alcoholic are cognitively impaired not only when high or drunk, but sometimes for many days or longer after their last use due to hormonal and neural changes that accompany addiction. Substance-dependent individuals have a responsibility to themselves, their families, and society to do everything in their power to achieve and maintain sobriety. Similarly, society has a responsibility to the substance-dependent individual to provide competent and effective treatment.

Robert H.: Chicken or the Egg

Robert H., referred to at the beginning of this chapter, is a fortyish-year-old man, married, with a young son and a daughter "in the oven." He had a promising business career and lives in an upper middle-class neighborhood. Robert drank a pint of vodka every day and sometimes more on the weekends. With two prior DUI's and prior court-ordered programs, he knew he had the disease of alcoholism, but has no idea how he became an alcoholic. The court programs he attended were punitive and not very instructive.

When he was growing up in a middle-class neighborhood on the East Coast, everybody drank. His father was German and loved his beer (everyday), and his mother was Spanish and had a taste for wine. Alcoholism was apparent for generations in both family trees. Robert had his first drink at fourteen years old—"normal" for his household and neighborhood.

Robert was also depressed most of the time. He saw several psychiatrists who diagnosed him as such. He was told by one doctor that it is difficult to distinguish depression from alcoholism. He was told it was a "chicken or the egg" situation—can't tell what caused what. He tried antidepressants, but nothing worked.

After the accident with his son, he went to a respected treatment facility for ninety days, where he learned he had a genetic predisposition to alcoholism. His "social drinking" induced changes in his brain that made him want more and more. He had no idea this could happen to him. A doctor at the center told him he had to stop drinking to see if his depression was due to the alcohol. The doctor told him the DSM-IV states that one cannot make the diagnosis of a mood disorder when there is concurrent substance abuse. He had to get sober first.

Robert had a common problem nicknamed the "twin demons of drinking and depression." His story is not unlike many who seek help for depression or other psychiatric illnesses while they are abusing mood-altering substances. Comorbid psychiatric illness and substance abuse are often difficult to untangle without skilled professional evaluation and treatment. *This is exactly why I strongly encourage the reader to seek individual professional advice for a mental health and/or substance problem.* Robert was lucky. Several of his ex-friends from the old neighborhood are dead.

Robert finished his treatment and stayed sober in AA. Today, four years later, Robert remains sober, with his health intact, although his wife divorced him and he had to find a new line of work. His son's leg healed quickly; however, their relationship is healing very slowly. Sober, Robert is no longer depressed and takes no medications. Today Robert is active in the program of Alcoholics Anonymous, going to meetings, working The Steps, and being of service. He is content. His son's injury still haunts him, and it likely will for life.

Chapter 2

Evolution of Addiction: Imaginary Darwinian Fitness through Mood-Altering Drugs

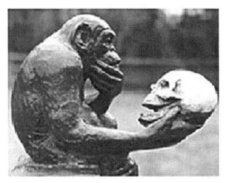

What went wrong?
(original photo by Hugo Rheinhold, 1892)

Possible Evolutionary Advantage of Drug Use In Ancient Civilization

With his book *The Origin of Species*, Charles Darwin offered two fundamental scientific postulates: The first suggests that all living things on earth are descendants of earlier species (i.e., evolution). The second suggests that natural selection is the architect of evolution. Natural selection drives evolution through adaptations to environmental challenges. Organisms that develop beneficial adaptations, increasing the likelihood that they will survive, are more likely to pass on these adaptive genes to their offspring than organisms that fail to develop beneficial adaptations. Consequently, over time, the organisms that fail to adapt and survive contribute fewer genes and become less prominent in a species. Although scientists and others often think about evolution with respect to physical changes among a species, the theory of evolution also can provide a unique perspective about behavioral processes that emerge within a species, such as addiction.

Humans, comprising the genus *Homo*, appeared between 1.5 and 2.5 million years ago, a time that roughly coincides with the start of the Pleistocene period 1.8 million years ago. Because the Pleistocene period ended a mere 12,000 years ago, most human adaptations either newly evolved during the Pleistocene period, or were maintained by stabilizing selection during the Pleistocene period (Gould, 1997). Evolutionary theory, therefore, proposes that the majority of human psychological mechanisms are adapted to increasing Darwinian fitness encountered in Pleistocene environments. In broad terms, these activities include those of growth and development, differentiation, maintenance, mating, parenting, and social relationships.

Drug addiction is not just a physiological reaction to a chemical but hypothesized to be a mode of psychological compensation for a decrease in Darwinian fitness (Panksepp, 2006; Hall, 2002). *Evolutionary theories suggest an intermediate and fleeting expected gain associated with drug addiction correlated with the conservation in humans of archaic neural circuitry—the brain's primitive reward center (a. k. a. the mesolimbic dopamine system).*

Two products of evolution deserve special mention in the development of addiction in humans (Saah, 2005). First, the brain's *limbic system*, harboring the reward centers, can be traced back down the evolutionary tree to lizards and snakes (MacLean, 1990). The limbic reward centers function to reinforce important fitness-benefitting behaviors like eating, drinking, sleeping, and engaging in sex. Unfortunately, they are vulnerable to corruption. Many drugs of abuse mimic naturally occurring neurotransmitters that activate the brain's reward system, co-opting it for purposes not part of the original design (Hall, 2002). This ability to mimic natural neurotransmitters, in a mainly effortless but reliable way, can contribute to ongoing drug taking. Many addictionologists assert that this is why psychoactive drugs "commandeer" normal functions of the

35

reward system, in terminology coined by the psychologist, Hembolt, in 1902. A similar modern term chosen by this author is "hijack."

The neurochemical changes in the brain associated with reward/ punishment tests of fitness and viability are perceived by mammals as emotions, and emotions drive human behavior. The emotions perceived by humans after drug ingestion either improve upon our positive affective emotions, or reduce emotions of negative affect (Cooper, 1995). We feel more fit, in Darwinian terms. Most often, this psychological perception of increased viability is false (Panksepp, 2002, 2006).

Second, most addiction involves ingesting, in some way, plant-related substances. The existence of these substances probably emerged, however, not to promote other species to consume plants, but to prevent predatory species from consuming plants. Evolutionary biologists point out that animals, including man, ingesting mind-altering substances might be a method of defense and a way to ensure their safety (Nesse, 1997, 2002). Ironically, the natural toxins, which deter some predators from consuming these plants, have served as temptations for humans, who discovered, and find attractive, their psychoactive properties. The evolutionary development of the brain's reward system and the evolutionary development of defense toxins in plants were likely independent; however, the interaction of these consequents of evolution seems to have created the opportunity for addiction.

Evolution of the Human Brain

By the time the first vertebrates and fish began to swim the oceans, around 500 million years ago, the first primitive lobes of the brain had also become fashioned through the progressive collectivization of primitive neural ganglia (small collection of nerve cells). This included the olfactory-limbic lobe (the forebrain), which was concerned with the detection of olfactory/pheromone chemicals that might belay the presence of a predator, prey, or a mate; the optic lobe of the midbrain visual apparatus, which was responsive to visual messages; and the hindbrain, which was concerned with movement. By 450,000 years ago, the first sharks had acquired a limbic system, which they, like modern humans, still possess today. Throughout its evolution, the human brain has acquired three components that progressively appeared and became superimposed: the oldest, located deep and to the back; the next one, resting on an intermediate position; and the most recent, situated on top and to the front. They are aptly described by renowned neuroscientist Paul MacLean (1990) as the *"triune brain."*

First, the *archipallium,* or primitive (reptilian) brain, comprises the structures of the brain stem (medulla, pons, cerebellum), the lower midbrain, the lower portions of the motor system, and the olfactory bulbs. It corresponds to the *reptile brain,* also called *"R-complex,"* by Dr. MacLean. The term derives from the fact that comparative neuroanatomists once believed that the forebrains of reptiles and birds were dominated by these structures. Parts of the reward centers are stationed in the archipallium.

Second, the *paleopallium,* or intermediate brain, comprises the structures of the *limbic system.* The limbic system is present in higher-order reptiles, fish (sharks), and inferior mammals and is often referred to as the *"reward center"* of the brain because of its rich dopaminergic innervations and numerous nuclei. The limbic system is also called the *"old mammalian"* or *"paleomammalian"* brain. The old mammalian brain consists of the septum, amygdala, hypothalamus, hippocampal complex, and cingulate cortex. MacLean first introduced the term *"limbic system"* to refer to this set of interconnected brain structures in a paper in 1952. Whatever the merits of the triune brain hypothesis, MacLean's recognition of the limbic system as a major functional system in the brain has won wide acceptance among neuroscientists, and it is generally regarded as his most important contribution to the field.

Third, the *neopallium,* also known as the superior or rational (new mammalian) brain, comprises almost the whole of the hemispheres (made up of a more recent type of cortex, called *neocortex*) and some subcortical neuronal groups. It corresponds to the brain of the superior mammals, thus including the primates and, consequently, the human brain. The neocortex is unique to mammals.

According to MacLean, the three subsets of the brain may be likened to three biological computers that, although interconnected, retain *"their peculiar types of intelligence, subjectivity, sense of time and space, memory, mobility and other less specific functions."*

Triune Brain

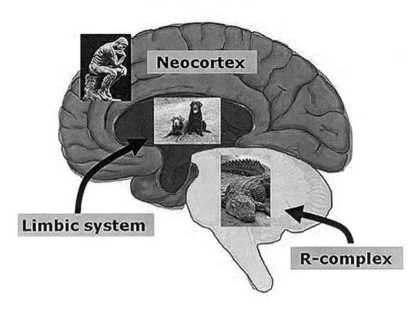

The primitive brain, or R-complex, is responsible for self-preservation. In the R-complex occur the instinctive reactions of the so-called reflex arcs and the commands that allow some involuntary actions and the control of certain visceral functions (cardiac, pulmonary, intestinal, etc.), indispensable to the preservation of life. The development of the olfactory bulbs and their connections made possible an accurate analysis of olfactory stimuli and the improvement of answers oriented by odors, such as approach, attack, flight, and mating. MacLean contended that the reptilian complex was responsible for species-typical instinctual behaviors involved in aggression, dominance, territoriality, and ritual displays. It is there that the mechanisms of aggression and repetitive behavior develop. It is also in the R-complex that the first manifestations of the phenomena of ritualism started—the animal tries to define its hierarchical position inside the group and establish its own space in the ecological niche. Throughout evolution, some of these reptilian functions were lost or minimized. In humans, the amygdala and the entorhinal (olfactory) cortex are the only limbic structures that connect with the R-complex.

In 1878, the French neurologist Paul Broca discovered an area containing several nuclei of grey matter (neurons) on the medial surface of the mammalian brain, immediately underneath the cortex, which he denominated the limbic lobe (from the Latin word *"limbus"* that implies the idea of circle, ring, surrounding, etc.) since it forms a kind of border around the brain stem (Panksepp, 1998). Years later (1949), the entirety of these structures would receive the name of *"limbic system"* by Paul MacLean. The limbic system developed with the emergence of the inferior (primitive) mammals. This system commands certain behaviors that are necessary for the survival of all mammals. It gives rise and modulates specific functions that allow the animal to distinguish between the agreeable and the disagreeable. Here specific affective (emotional) functions are developed, such as the one that induces the females to nurse and protect their toddlers, or the one that induces these animals to develop ludic behaviors (playful moods). *Emotions and feelings, such as wrath, fright, passion, love, hate, joy, and sadness, are mammalian inventions and originate in the limbic system.* The limbic system is also responsible for some aspects of personal identity and for important functions related to memory.

The physiological and behavioral features unique to mammals are in the limbic brain. The prototypical center of the limbic system—the hypothalamus, for example—is responsible for setting our temperature through manipulation of the animal's metabolic rate. Indeed, the hypothalamus is why we are warm-blooded. *As the center of emotions, the limbic system facilitates relationships.* Mammals, unlike reptiles and phylogenetically lower animals, care for their young. *Mammals evolved brains hardwired for mother-child and other relationships; that is, mammals are naturally social* (more in Chapter 9).

> *"The most common reaction a reptile has to its young is indifference; it lays its eggs and walks (or slithers) away. Mammals form close-knit, mutually nurturant social groups-families-in which members spend time touching and caring for one another. Parents nourish and safeguard their young, and each other, from the hostile world outside their group. A mammal will risk and sometimes lose its life to protect a child or mate from attack. A garter snake or salamander watches the death of its kin with an unblinking eye."*
>
> ~Thomas Lewis, 2000

When the superior mammals evolved, the highest order of the brain developed the *neopallium,* or *rational brain.* The neopallium is a highly complex net of neural cells capable of producing symbolic language, thus enabling man to exercise skillful intellectual tasks, such as reading, writing, and performing mathematical calculations. The neopallium is the great generator of ideas or, as expressed by Paul MacLean, *"it is the mother of invention and the father of abstractive thought."* The *cerebral cortex* (neocortex) is the newest, outermost area of our brain. The oldest mammals (e.g., opossums) have only a thin layer of cerebral cortex. Rabbits have a little more, cats a bit more, etc. Monkeys have a substantial cerebral cortex. Humans, and only humans, have an enormous cerebral cortex.

Remarkably, however, the human reptilian brain (R-complex) and limbic system are similar in size and structure to phylogenetically inferior animals. Indeed, our ancestors evolved a huge cerebral cortex, while the older brain areas did not change. The cerebral cortex learns new things. Animals with a cerebral cortex can find new foods, survive in new environments, or change their mating tactics to improve reproductive success. The human cerebral cortex goes beyond learning new foods and survival skills. Our brains can think in abstractions. We communicate via symbols (e.g., language), consider the past and future, and sacrifice our personal interests not only for our families (as other mammals do) but also for ideas (e.g., honor and country).

These three cerebral layers appear, one after the other, during the development of the embryo and the fetus (ontogenesis), recapitulating, chronologically, the evolution of animal species (phylogenesis), from the lizards up to the Homo sapiens (Nesse, 1990). In biology, there is a saying: *"Ontogeny recapitulates phylogeny."* A child's development mimics its species' evolution. Infants live in their reptilian brains. They eat, breathe, crawl, sleep, etc. Children live in their limbic brains. They feel emotions strongly. They use emotions to form relationships. Adolescents live in their cerebral cortexes. They strive to become unique individuals. They quest to find abstract principles to live by. Adult relationships invert childhood development. Men and women use cerebral cortex abstractions (e.g., gender roles) to attract opposite sex partners. If a couple then feels "limbic-brain" emotionally connected "chemistry," they form a relationship. If the relationship goes well, eventually they are in bed, using their old-mammalian and reptilian brains. (Life is grand, indeed.)

The Evolutionary Advantage of Emotion

The evolution of the limbic system brought about indicators of levels of fitness in the form of chemical signals perceived as emotion (Panksepp, 2002; LeDoux, 1995 & 1996). In simple terms, the limbic system is made of neurons that release chemicals when stimulated, and this release leads to subjective feelings of well being or distress in response to stimuli (Buss, 2000). Around the world, people recognize that humans experience transient alterations of subjective state in response to information. People also agree that these alterations are often (with varying degrees of voluntary control) outwardly expressed, they motivate action, and they involve a change in one's perception of oneself, one's surroundings, and one's goals. English speakers label these experiences *"emotions,"* and similar terms occur in many languages. Because the constituents of this category vary across languages, some anthropologists argue that emotions are primarily cultural in nature, and are incommensurate across cultures. However, critics of this position note that, while labels and connotations differ across cultures, many emotional expressions (particularly those involving the face) are easily recognized by outsiders, and outsiders learn to map local labels onto their own emotion lexicon. *This suggests that—while cultures may determine the meaning of events that elicit emotions, and while cultures may glorify, disparage, ignore, or combine particular aspects of the emotion repertoire—the core aspects of human emotions are species-typical and, hence, likely to be the products of selection.*

In 1872, Darwin published *The Expression of the Emotions in Man and Animals* in which he presented evidence that some emotional expressions are recognizable across cultures and appear spontaneously in children (Gould, 1997). Darwin used the similarities between these expressions and those seen in animals to argue for common descent. While this perspective defied the Western tradition at the time, Darwin conformed to that tradition in viewing emotions' effects on reasoning as detrimental, describing human emotions as vestiges of earlier evolutionary stages in which the intellect was of less importance. Evolutionary psychologists seek to explain the influences of emotions on attention, memory, motivation, and other functions in terms of the recurrent challenges that have confronted humans.

The term "emotion" is derived from the Latin *emovere*, which means, literally, "to move." Emotionality, basically, is protective in function, and is closely related to movement and action. It promotes either survival of the individual through fight-or-flight responses or survival of the species through reproductive or social cooperative responses (Newlin, 2002). These emotions help direct physiology and behavior of an individual toward increasing Darwinian fitness. They essentially were tools chosen for the mechanisms of natural selection. *Positive emotions, such as euphoria and excitation, motivate toward increased gain and fitness states, whereas negative emotions—for instance, anxiety and pain—evolved as defenses for avoiding potential threats to fitness.*

The mammalian drive to escape danger is fueled by a capacity to feel negative emotions (Nesse, 2002). Negative emotions (pain, fear, stress, anxiety, etc.) have evolved in mammals to elude danger. Negative emotions are excellent defenses. If suppressed, we may find ourselves unarmed and unprepared to deal with problems much more detrimental than the original warning emotions. Those individuals that lack the capacity to suffer negative emotions, including the inability to experience physical pain, are unable to put up basic physiological and behavioral defenses and often find themselves dying at relatively young ages.

Mood-altering substances stimulate the limbic system by inducing positive emotions and a sense of well-being and placating negative emotions. This is why substance users experience feelings of pleasure, or "high," when they use them. Negative emotions, such as fear and anxiety, are reduced. *When mood-altering substances are used, they may hijack the brain's limbic system and emotions, promoting drug use to the exclusion of other adaptive activities.* The positive emotions and feelings of reproduction or eating are replaced by the "high" produced by the drug of choice. Since behaviors necessary for survival are displaced by drug use, the very life of organism is at risk.

Emotions in Animals

Charles Darwin's well-accepted ideas about evolutionary continuity contend that differences among species are differences in degree rather than kind. *All mammals (including humans) share neuroanatomical structures that are responsible for feelings, such as the amygdala and neurochemical pathways in the limbic system.* Axioms of evolutionary theory argue strongly for the presence of animal emotions, empathy, and moral behavior. Continuity allows us to connect the "evolutionary dots" among different species to highlight similarities in evolved traits, including individual feelings and passions.

Recent work in the areas of ethics and sociobiology suggests that it is philosophically legitimate to ascribe emotions to non-human animals (Moussaieff, 1996). Furthermore, it is sometimes argued that emotionality is a morally relevant psychological state shared by humans and non-humans. Psychologist Jaak Panksepp argues that rather than being a recent development of the human neo-cortex, the roots of consciousness (he uses the term "affective consciousness" to reflect its internal "feeling") can be traced right back to early mammals in deep ancient sub-neocortical limbic regions of the brain (Panksepp, 2005b, 2005c). Panksepp and his colleagues have identified seven basic emotional systems in mammals: seeking, rage, fear, lust, care, panic, and play. The human neocortex, in all its cognitive complexity, further processes these primary affects into more elaborate emotions, such as love, shame and empathy. The evidence for these core emotional systems is laid out in detail elsewhere (e.g., Panksepp, 2005b, 2005c), but here is a summary:

Areas of the brain that generate positive and negative affective states in humans and animals when electrically stimulated are remarkably similar, and the most powerful "feelings" are generated in deep, subcortical areas of the limbic system. The anatomy and neurochemistry of the limbic system and related subcortical areas are remarkably similar in all mammals and clearly evolutionarily homologous. Opiate and dopamine agonists are drugs of abuse in humans and also attractive to other mammals. PET studies show remarkable similarities in basic emotions in humans and other mammals, and these emotions arise in deep, subcortical areas of the brain (McMillan, 2001; Watt, 2005).

A basic rule of survival is to approach food sources and potential mates (appetitive stimuli), and avoid danger, such as predators (aversive stimuli). These functions are programmed into the limbic and reward centers of the mammalian brain. External stimuli provoke emotional or motivational states that are processed primarily by the core of the emotional brain. The structures of the core circuits are highly conserved across species, but component neurons are often tuned to stimuli with species-specific significance (e.g., odors of predators, pheromones, etc). When an animal learns to perform an arbitrary response to approach or avoid a stimulus, natural selection cannot hard-wire connections between receptor and response mechanisms for every single experience (Rolls,

1999). For example, suppose a rat learns that turning in a right-hand circle gives it food and turning in a left-hand circle gives it an electric shock and then, when the experimenter changes the rules of the experiment, learns to go left to get food and right to avoid a shock. Natural selection could not have led to the evolution of rats able to do this by complex rules, or complex higher cortical wiring.

The only way the rat could achieve such a feat would be by having a *simple reward-punishment system* that allowed it to associate any action that happened to make it "feel better" or "feel worse" and either repeat or avoid such actions in the future (Rolls, 1999). Specific rules (such as always turning right or always turning toward red stimuli) would be very much less effective than more general rules (repeat what leads to feeling better or pleasure). General emotional states of pleasure and suffering would enable animals to exploit many more behavioral strategies to increase their fitness than specific stimulus-response links.

Without emotions to guide it, an animal would have no way of knowing whether a behavior never performed before by any of its ancestors should be repeated or not. By monitoring the consequences of its behavior by whether it leads to "pleasure" or "suffering," it can build up a complex string of quite arbitrary responses. It can learn, for example, that pressing a lever leads to the appearance of a striped box that contains food. By finding the striped box "pleasurable," because it is associated with food, and learning to press the lever to obtain this pleasure, the rat learns to obtain food through a route that is not open to an animal totally pre-programmed in its responses. Emotions are, therefore, necessary to reinforcement learning.

Pavlovian conditioning in primates suggests similar mechanisms supporting this basic form of emotional learning (Savage-Rumbaugh, 1994). The main difference might be that emotional processing from the core structures radiates in primates to a larger array of partially or fully neocortical structures that re-process emotion and link it to memory, planning, and decision making. The essential difference derives from the major role of social stimuli to elicit emotions in primates.

In primates, it is clear that the majority of emotional states are centered on social interactions, because in almost all primate species, individuals live within elaborate social dominance hierarchies. Here, appropriate responses to members of the group can reduce the threat of attack or increase access to food, reproductive partners, or allies that indirectly reduce threats and increase access to rewards. Indeed, the majority of emotional states in such primate species occur during social interactions. These socio-emotional interactions depend on the identity and dominance status of the participants, as well as on the recent history of aggression/affiliation and, perhaps most critically, reproductive success (Panksepp, 1998).

Primates—in particular, great apes—are candidates for highly developed capabilities for empathy and theories of mind (knowing what the other is thinking). This has allowed primates to develop highly complex social systems. Young apes and their mothers have very strong bonds of attachment. Often when a baby chimpanzee or gorilla dies, the mother will carry the body around for several days (McHenry, 2009), Jane Goodall has described chimpanzees as exhibiting mournful behavior. See notably the example of the gorilla Koko, who expressed sadness over the death of her pet cat, All Ball.

> *"All Ball" was a pet cat of Koko, the famous gorilla living in Woodside, California, who is purported to communicate via sign language. One day All Ball escaped from Koko's cage and was hit and killed by a car. Later, Koko's trainer claimed that when she signed to Koko that All Ball had gone, Koko signed "Bad, sad-bad" and "Frown cry-frown sad." The trainer also reported later hearing Koko making a sound akin to human weeping. In 1985, Koko was allowed to pick out two new kittens from a litter to be her companions. She cared for the kittens as if they were her young."*
> ~Dr. Francine Patterson, psychologist, sociobiologist, 1987

Dr. Patterson uses Koko's story, and many others, to argue that non-human species can have human-like emotions. Research suggests that canines can experience an array of positive and negative emotions in a similar manner to people. The existence and nature of personality traits in dogs have been studied (15,329 dogs of 164 different breeds) and five consistent and stable "narrow traits" identified, described as playfulness, curiosity/fearlessness, chase-proneness, sociability and aggressiveness. A further higher order axis for shyness–boldness was also identified (Svartberga, 2004). Psychology research has shown that human faces are asymmetrical with the gaze instinctively moving to the right side of a face upon encountering other humans to obtain information about

45

their emotions and state (Guo, 2007). Recent research at the University of Lincoln shows that dogs share this instinct when meeting a human being, and only when meeting a human being (i.e., not other animals or other dogs). As such, they are the only non-primate species known to do so (Alleyne, 2008).

The emotions of cats have also been studied scientifically for many years. It has been shown that cats can learn to manipulate their owners through vocalizations that are similar to the cries of human babies. Some cats learn to add a purr to the cry, which makes it less harmonious to humans and, therefore, harder to ignore. Individual cats learn to make these cries through operant conditioning; when a particular cry elicits a positive response from a human, the cat is more likely to use that cry in the future (McComb, 2009).

Emotions in Humans

In 1872, Darwin published *The Expression of the Emotions in Man and Animals* in which he presented evidence that all humans, and even other animals, show emotion through remarkably similar behaviors. For Darwin, emotion had an evolutionary history that could be traced across cultures and species-an unpopular view at the time. Today, many psychologists agree that certain emotions are universal to all humans, regardless of culture: anger, fear, surprise, disgust, happiness, and sadness. In writing Expression, Darwin corresponded with numerous researchers, including French physician Guillaume-Benjamin-Amand Duchenne, who believed that human faces expressed at least sixty discrete emotions, each of which depended on its own dedicated group of facial muscles. In contrast, Darwin thought the facial muscles worked together to create a core set of just a few emotions.

Duchenne studied emotion by applying electrical currents to the faces of his subjects, sending their muscles into a state of continual contraction (Freitas-Magalhaes, 2009). By stimulating the right combination of facial muscles, Duchenne mimicked genuine emotional expression. He produced more than sixty photographic plates of his subjects demonstrating what he believed were distinct emotions. But Darwin disagreed and was quoted as saying, "I don't believe this. This isn't true."

Darwin hypothesized that only some of Duchenne's slides represented universal human emotions. To test this idea, he arranged a single-blind study at his home in Kent County, England. Darwin chose eleven of Duchenne's slides, placed them in a random order, and presented them one at a time to over twenty of his guests without any hints or leading questions. He then asked his friends to guess which emotion each slide represented and tabulated their answers. That kind of experimental control would be considered deeply flawed today, but it was progressive for Darwin's time. According to the handwritten notes and data tables, Darwin's guests agreed almost unanimously about certain emotions—like happiness, sadness, fear, and surprise—but strongly disagreed about what other more ambiguous slides showed. For Darwin, only photographic slides that earned overwhelming agreement depicted one of the true universal human emotions. Darwin used the results of his nineteenth-century experiment to inform his own understanding of emotion and his writing of *Expression*. But his pioneering methods remain relevant to psychologists today.

Although there is no consensus as to the number of basic emotions, commonly proposed members include happiness, surprise, fear, sadness, anger, disgust, contempt, shame, and guilt. Emotional terms are often thematically linked; that is, terms such as "terror," "fear," and "anxiety" all revolve around a single core experience. Furthermore, these core experiences are often associated with readily recognizable facial expressions. This has led many psychologists to propose the existence of discrete basic emotions; it is thought that the full panoply of emotions is generated from these unitary, elementary constituents through processes of combination of basic emotions and/or fine cultural discrimination. *At the most rudimentary level, emotions can be broken down into "good" (happiness, love, etc.) and "bad" (fear, anger, etc.); an event, interaction or situation elicits either an appetitive (want more) or aversive (want less) response.* Our limbic reward centers dictate these rudimentary responses, which are *evolutionarily adaptive*.

Actual cognitive appraisal of emotions in humans is, of course, much more diverse due to the interaction between our limbic reward systems and extremely large neocortical centers (LeDoux, 1996, Panksepp, 2006). For example, rather than discussing a single emotion—fear, which is a response to imminent danger—evolutionary psychologists predict the existence of multiple types of fear, each associated with such distinct classes of threats as predators, rival con-specifics, social exclusion, snakes, spiders, etc. Further subdivisions may occur on the basis of context. Activation of a given emotion—say, fear of predators in the twilight—directs attention to relevant information (potential signs of predators), sharpens sensory modalities relevant to that information (visual, auditory, etc.), cues patterns of interpretation (ambiguous shadows look like predators, etc.), readies relevant motor patterns (fight-or-flight), reassigns priority among goals (escape versus feeding, mating, playing chess, etc.), searches relevant memory categories (information about predators), and so on. Nonetheless, in all contexts, the emotion of "fear" is adaptive.

Anger in response to having been cheated is adaptive, because it decreases the likelihood of future defections against oneself, particularly if it is disproportionate in relation to the transgression. Because disproportionate response is costly, an auxiliary mechanism is necessary to impel aggression, and anger serves this purpose. Similarly, because gratitude in response to generosity motivates reciprocation, individuals who feel gratitude avoid the short-term gain reaped by defection and obtain the long-term gain provided by cooperation. Hirshleifer (1987) suggests that the advantages of anger and gratitude are not limited to reciprocal exchanges but pertain in any situation of potential cooperation.

Many authors propose that guilt evolved in order to (1) dissuade individuals from harming beneficial relationships and/or (2) motivate them to repair damage done to such relationships (Rolls, 1999). One difficulty with these explanations is that, even granted the existence of cognitive biases, selection should favor the ability to cheat surreptitiously, yet guilt motivates reparation even when the transgression is undiscovered. In most cultures guilt creates *internal emotional stress* in the individual, which manifests itself in deleterious physiological responses; guilt and its incumbent stress, therefore, are evolutionarily *maladaptive*. Relief from guilt is evolutionarily *adaptive*. (More on stress in Chapter 5 and guilt in Chapter 7.)

Evolutionary theorists have noted that romantic love functions to commit individuals to a long-term cooperative mateship and signal that commitment to the partner—two valuable functions, given human infant dependence on adults for survival (Buss, 2001). Love is adaptive. Romantic love exhibits a distinct chronology, with an initial period of obsessive ideation eventually giving way to a less intrusive form of attachment. The early phase may both strongly dissuade defection during a period of scrutiny and motivate energetic signaling of commitment. Once a cooperative enterprise has been established, the costs of the mating enterprise are appraised and the necessary emotional intensity reduced on both counts.

Love is closely tied to jealousy. Evolutionary psychologists examine emotions such as jealousy, in light of recurrent adaptive challenges. For example, the evolutionary psychologist, David Buss (2000), notes that a principal hazard for men is misdirected investment due to promiscuity, while a principal hazard for women is cessation of male provisioning due to abandonment. Consistent with these observations, Buss finds that men are more disturbed by the prospect of a mate's sexual infidelity, while women are more disturbed by the prospect of a mate's emotional attachment to rival women.

While human emotions are clearly derived from a psychological foundation shared by social mammals, we likely possess some emotions that are considerably less developed, or wholly absent, in other creatures (Cosmides, 1997). Humans are unique in the extent of their reliance on socially transmitted information in coping with physical and social environments. An important class of emotions consists of those that mediate the acquisition, use, and dissemination of cultural information. Admiration of successful persons involves a desire for proximity and a willingness to provide client services to obtain it, as well as a desire for close observation and imitation. These patterns lead individuals to adopt ideas and practices of social utility. (More on man's instinct for social interaction, beyond courtship, in Chapter 9.)

Plant-Derived Psychoactive Drugs

Drugs of abuse are nearly all derived from, or based on the molecular structure of, plant products. Psychoactive drugs have their actions via their molecular similarities with endogenous neurotransmitters. The fact that plants produce chemicals so similar to our own brain chemicals is likely to be the product of co-evolution. One possible scenario is that addictive drugs are produced by plants as neurotoxins, functioning to reduce predation (Nesse, 1997). For example, the wabayo tree produces ouabain, a chemical that causes neurons to lose polarity and fail to fire, causing confusion and death (Nesse, 2002).

Alternatively, a mutually beneficial co-evolutionary relationship might exist between animals and addictive drug-producing plants. Sullivan and

Hegen (2002) argue that drug seeking might actually be adaptive to humans in that drugs, like other plants, are essentially food. Since psychoactive drugs are similar chemically to neurotransmitters, they are supposedly easily metabolized into neurotransmitter precursors, otherwise attained in a more energy-inefficient manner through other foods. Essentially, plant drugs are vitamin supplements. Presumably, the plants benefit from this proposed relationship in that their seeds are sewn by way of the human's digestive tract (or even intentionally by humans with gardens). Indeed, psychoactive plants are widely cultivated today, suggesting that their production of drugs has lent them reproductive success.

Many psychotropic plants evolved to react with the host animal's brain to deter threats from herbivores and pathogenic invasions. These are called "allelochemical" responses and evolved to imitate mammalian neurotransmitters so as to act as competitive binders and obstruct normal nervous system functioning. The allelochemical neurotransmitter analogs were not anciently as potent as forms of abused substances used in modern environments, but instead were milder precursors that had an impact on the development of the mammalian central nervous system (Saah, 2005). The fit of allelochemicals within the central nervous system indicates some co-evolutionary activity between mammalian brains and psychotropic plants, meaning they interacted ecologically and therefore responded to one another evolutionarily. Basically, a series of changes occurred between the mammalian brain and psychotropic plants allowing them to affect one another during their evolution. This would have been possible only with mammalian central nervous system exposure to these allelochemicals— therefore to ancient mammalian psychotropic substance use. The evidence for this theory is compelling. For example, the mammalian brain has evolved receptor systems for plant substances, such as the certain opioids, which are not produced by the mammalian body itself. The mammalian body has also evolved to develop defenses against over toxicity, such as exogenous substance metabolism and vomiting reflexes.

It is likely that the co-evolutionary relationships between animals and psychoactive plants have evolved with different drugs. For example, it seems likely that plant production of cocaine and nicotine—which are present in plant tissues necessary for life, such as leaves—evolved as toxins designed to reduce predation by animals. Opium, on the other hand, is stored in pods housing ripe seeds, suggesting that this drug provides an incentive for eating (and distributing) seeds, just as sweet fruit does for other plants. Likewise, marijuana primarily stores psychoactive compounds in seed-containing flower structures.

Psychoactive Drug Use in Animals

Given the vast similarities between the human and animal mesolimbic brain, it should not be surprising that animals seek alterations in their emotional states through mood-altering substances (Samorini, 2002). Samorini recounts how birds in the Western United States, high on the fermented berries of the California Holly, engage in drunken orgies. It is well known that cats get high on catnip, an herb that gives male cats spontaneous erections and makes female cats adopt mating stances. In his book, Samorini reveals how mandrills in Gabon, Africa, dig up and eat the roots of the powerfully hallucinogenic Iboga Tabernanthe to prepare for combat to claim a female. The reader learns that, around the world, psychedelic-facilitated animal orgies facilitate the continuation of many species.

According to accounts in Samorini's book, the vervet monkey has long been known to have a taste for alcoholic beverages, or at least their mood-altering properties. In experiments on the Caribbean island of Saint Kitts, scientists have found that their drinking patterns are curiously human. Given the choice of whether to drink or not, 15 percent of the vervets stay abstinent. Most of them are moderate, social drinkers who like their alcohol diluted with fruit juice. About 15 per cent drink heavily. They gulp booze down, pass out, and do it all over again the same day, as well as day after day. Some intoxicated monkeys get aggressive, some get amorous, others think everything is funny, and some get grumpy. The monkeys are the descendants of animals introduced as pets in the seventeenth century. They lived wild, but people who wanted to eat the monkeys discovered they could trap them by leaving out sweetened rum in coconut shells. The monkeys drank the rum, passed out, and were later eaten—maladaptive, to say the least. Today the monkeys occasionally raid local bars in search of rum. Scientists hope genetic studies of the monkeys could help pinpoint genes that make some of us prone to alcoholism.

Cats enjoy the mood-altering qualities of a plant called catmint or catnip, *Nepeta cataria*, a member of the mint family. It makes domestic cats—and even some wild cats like cougars, lions and lynx—exhibit bizarre behaviors. They sniff, lick, and chew it, shaking their heads, rolling around and drooling, and generally going nuts for about fifteen minutes. Then the effect wears off. Cats seem to "reset" after a couple of hours, and then do it again. The volatile chemical in the herb that causes the reaction is nepetalactone, a member of the terpene group that also includes turpentine. No one knows precisely what effect nepetalactone has on a cat's brain, but it may stimulate the regions that control sex, appetite, and mood. A third of domestic cats do not react to catnip at all, however. In order to sense the chemical, they need to have a certain gene that gives them a nepetalactone receptor in their *vomeronasal* organ, a structure found above the feline palate that detects pheromones.

Cats in Japan like a different drug, the leaves of the matatabi plant, which contains compounds similar to nepetalactone. But it causes a different behavior, making them lie on their backs with their paws in the air. In people, catnip can act as a mild stimulant or as a mild sedative. Some people swear that catnip tea helps them sleep, while catnip supplements are marketed as remedies for migraines. However, one possible side effect is, unforgivingly, a headache.

Elephants have long been notorious for their passion for alcohol. African elephants can become extremely excitable and aggressive when they eat the fermenting fruit of several types of palm trees. Their Asian cousins are more raucous, regularly killing people and destroying homes in drunken stampedes. It has been reported, for instance, that elephants stumbled across casks of homemade rice beer after destroying granaries in search of food in the northeastern state of Assam. They broke the casks, downed the beer, and then trampled at least six people to death. The problem seems to be getting worse, because the numbers of elephants have increased in the region since the Assam government put a ban on hunting around twenty years ago. At the same time, the elephants' habitat has been shrinking due to deforestation and development. Every winter, conservation groups hear reports of drunken birds slamming into windows or plummeting to their deaths from buildings and trees. The drunks are most commonly robins, followed by cedar waxwings.

Lapland reindeer had a taste for hallucinogenic mushrooms. Ian Darwin Edwards of Scotland's Royal Botanic Garden in Edinburgh, who researches the use of plants by the Sami people of Lapland, reported that there is good historical evidence that shamans of northern European tribes used mushrooms to induce hallucinations as part of rituals and healing (Samorini, 2002). Their fungus of choice was probably the fly agaric mushroom, *Amanita muscaria*, a red mushroom with white spots that often appears in fairy-tale books, and it is common in northern birch forests. According to historical records, the shaman people fed the mushrooms to reindeer and collected their urine. The shaman would drink it, and then other people would drink their urine. The hallucinogenic drugs in fly agaric can be passed on through urine in a more refined form, according to Edwards. The mushrooms contain the toxin muscimol, which is structurally similar to the neurotransmitter gamma-aminobutyric acid (GABA) and competes with it for binding sites in the brain. Muscimol induces hallucinations.

Psychoactive Drug Use in Ancient Cultures

Drug use is a practice that dates to prehistoric times. There is archaeological evidence of the use of psychoactive substances dating back at least 10,000 years, and historical evidence of cultural use over the past 5,000 years (Stringer, 1994). While medicinal use seems to have played a very large role, it has been suggested that the urge to alter one's consciousness is a primary human desire, akin to sex (McHenry, 2009). Several primitive civilizations use psychotropic plants as entheogens (to find God). The long history of drug use in ancient cultures and even children's desire for spinning, swinging, or sliding indicate that the drive to alter one's state of mind is universal human phenomenon.

Archaeological records indicate the presence of psychotropic plants and drug use in ancient civilizations as far back as early hominid species 200 million years ago (Sullivan, 2002, Saah, 2005). Approximately 13,000 years ago, Timor natives used betel nut (Areca catechu), as did natives in Thailand around 10,700 years ago. At the beginning of European colonialism, and perhaps for 40,000 years before that, Australian aborigines were noted to use nicotine from two different indigenous sources: pituri plant (Duboisia hopwoodii) and Nicotiana gossel. North and South Americans also used nicotine from their indigenous plants N. tabacum and N. rustica. Ethiopians and Northern Africans had found an ephedrine-analog, khat (Catha edulis), before European colonization. Cocaine (Erythroxylum coca) was ingested by Ecuadorians about 5,000 years ago and by the indigenous people of the Western Andes almost 7,000 years. It is reported that the substances were popularly administered through the buccal cavity within the cheek. Although the buccal method is believed to be the most standard method of drug administration, inhabitants of the Americas may have also administered substances nasally, rectally, and by smoking.

It is hypothesized that ancient civilizations had a view of psychotropic plants as food sources, not as external chemicals altering internal homeostasis or mood (Sullivan, 2002). The perceived effects by these groups of drugs were tolerance to thermal fluctuations, increased energy, and decreased fatigue, all advantageous to *fitness* by allowing longer foraging sessions as well as a greater ability to sustain in times of limited resources. The plants were used as nutritional sources providing vitamins, minerals, and proteins rather than recreational psychotropic substances inducing inebriation. Therefore, drug-containing plants became food sources to prevent decreased fitness from starvation and death. It is believed that early hominid species evolved in conjunction with the psychotropic flora due to constant exposure to one another. This may be what eventually allowed the above civilizations to use the flora as nutritional substances, therefore increasing both their fitness and viability.

Hallucinogenic drugs are among the oldest drugs used by humankind, as hallucinogens naturally occur in mushrooms, cacti, and various other plants. Whether the use of hallucinogens is encouraged, unregulated, regulated, or prohibited, and whether hallucinogens are used for recreational, medicinal, or spiritual purposes, varies from culture to culture and nation to nation. Hallucinogen use is relatively rare in most current societies. In most countries of the world, common hallucinogens are illegal, and their possession is considered a crime as of 2003. Rarely, an exception will be made for religious purposes. For example, in the United States, possession of peyote cactus is illegal for most purposes, but the cactus is legally grown and used for religious rituals among various Southwestern Native American tribes (El-Seedi, 2005).

In contrast to most modern societies, many tribal societies actively encourage the use of hallucinogens, usually as part of a religious ritual. In some other tribes, it is tolerated and not seen as uncommon. Many sects of Christianity have associated hallucinogenic drug use with witches and the devil. Rumors circulated among medieval Europeans that the hallucinogen belladonna was a key ingredient of various magical flying ointments (Samorini, 2002). When applied to mucous membranes, alkaloids in the plant induce (among other effects) hallucinations, nausea, and a sensation of flying. Witches were commonly believed to fly through the air on broomsticks after using the ointment. Consequently, any association with the belladonna plant could have proven extremely dangerous and led to one's execution as a practitioner of witchcraft. Peyote cactus has been used in various Native American religious practices in the Southwestern United States and Mexico since long before Europeans arrived. The "ghost dance" religion that developed in the 1880s among Native Americans in the region involved peyote use. Rain forest tribes in the Amazon River basin have been known to make use of various hallucinogenic plants, as well.

An entheogen—"God inside us," in the strict sense—is a psychoactive substance used in a psychotherapeutic, religious, shamanic, or spiritual context. Historically, entheogens were mostly derived from plant sources and have been used in a variety of traditional religious contexts. Most entheogens do not produce drug dependency. With the advent of organic chemistry, many synthetic substances with similar psychoactive properties have been developed. Entheogens can supplement many diverse practices for healing, transcendence, and revelation, including: meditation, psychonautics, art projects, and psychedelic therapy.

Entheogens have been used in a ritualized context for thousands of years; their religious significance is well established in anthropological and modern evidences. Examples of traditional entheogens include: kykeon, ambrosia, iboga, soma, peyote, bufotenine, and ayahuasca (entheogens. org). Other traditional entheogens include cannabis, ethanol, ergine, psilocybe mushrooms, and opium. Many pure active compounds with psychoactive properties have been isolated from organisms and chemically synthesized, including LSD, mescaline, psilocin/psilocybin, DMT, salvinorin A, and ibogaine. Entheogens may be compounded through the work of a shaman or apothecary in a tea, admixture, or potion, like ayahuasca or bhang. Essentially all psychoactive drugs that are naturally occurring in plants, fungi, or animals, can be used in an entheogenic context or with entheogenic intent. Since non-psychoactive drugs can also be used in this type of context, the term "entheogen" refers primarily to substances that have been categorized based on their historical use.

Effect of Psychoactive Drugs on Emotions: Imaginary "Fitness"

"Psychoactive drugs induce emotions that at one point in mammalian evolutionary history signaled increased fitness, not happiness" (Nesse, 1997). In ancient environments positive emotions correlated with a sign of

increased fitness, such as successful foraging sessions or successful breeding. Mammals would feel euphoric only during times where fitness levels were high, the euphoria being indicative of survival and not a superfluous feeling of "happiness." Mammals would otherwise feel negative emotions when fitness levels were low. The effect of many psychoactive substances provided the same euphoric feeling, and may have had some increasing effects on fitness levels in ancient mammalian species. However, drug use today does not carry the same predicted increases in fitness and, in fact, may act as a "pathogen" on neural circuitry. The pathological potential primarily related to the potency of modern psychoactive drugs. Yet, these same drugs continue to target archaic mechanisms of the brain with the intent of inducing positive emotion, essentially blocking many neurological defenses.

Drugs that stimulate positive emotion mediate incentive and motivation in the limbic reward system (Berridge, 1998). Modern drug addiction fundamentally indicates a false increase of fitness, leading to increasing drug abuse to continue gain, even if the gain is realized as being false. This is the quintessential paradox among drug addicts. The motivation toward gain begins to take precedence over adaptive behaviors among addicted individuals. Some stimuli that imitate increased fitness may become greater priorities than true adaptive stimuli necessary for increased fitness, such as food and sleep (Panksepp, 2002). Individuals can, in turn, decrease their fitness by ignoring necessary behaviors for survival and fitness and focusing on a false positive emotion. The appetite for a drug may also override the drive to consummate, causing a drastic decrease in viability. Their emotional systems are now concentrated on drug seeking rather than survival.

In modern humans, drugs that may block negative emotions may be more useful than the endurance of ancient warnings of harm, like pain and fever (Nesse, 1997). Certain drugs can aid in pathology treatment, and while negative emotions may have been entirely necessary for the survival of ancient mammals, they may no longer be exclusively indicative of nociceptive or otherwise harmful stimuli. Hypersensitivity of our bodies' defense mechanisms has evolved, leading to unnecessary negative emotions for non-nociceptive stimuli as preventative defense. When there is a threat towards an individual's fitness, the modern body often responds with several different warning signs, perhaps several different types of negative emotions (pain, fever, and hallucination, for example).

Therefore, blocking a few of the negative emotions will *ideally* not disrupt the message. I emphasize the word "ideally" for this is not always the case. Frequently, there are situations in which drugs that block these defenses, such as anxiolytics (drugs used to treat anxiety), may contribute to the decreases in fitness by temporarily removing small negative emotions but leaving the individual vulnerable to a much larger harm (Nesse, 1994).

Emotional disposition has shown to specifically correlate with problematic use of alcohol (Cooper, 1995). If the perceived emotion before alcohol consumption is negative, the individual most likely is drinking to cope, with less control over his/her own use. In the case of a positive disposition before consumption, the user is said to drink to enhance, with more greatly controlled use of the substance. Hence, the drinker has a sense of improved "fitness." Since alcohol consumption alters normally functioning cognitive processes, it does not prove to be equal or superior to evolutionarily superior internal coping mechanisms.

The possibility that susceptibility to drug addiction enhances reproductive success, even at the expense of our health, may contribute to our present addictability. For example, if drug use in the evolutionary environment enhanced fitness (either through advantageous subjective effects, like alertness, etc., or by providing scarce nutritional resources), a preference for drugs might have been evolutionarily selected for, even if such a preference had long-term health consequences. For example, suppose chewing coca made one a great dancer, which enhanced social status and reproductive success in an evolutionary environment. A preference for coca might still evolve, even if coca also led to deadly mouth cancer in old age.

Additionally, some have argued that mesolimbic dopamine actually monitors opportunities for, and threatens one's reproductive success (Newlin, 2002; Panksepp, 2002). If drugs, for whatever reason, signal a huge fitness gain, compulsive self-administration could develop at the expense of personal health. An analogy of this could be electrical stimulation of certain mesolimbic brain areas, which are readily and compulsively self-administered by animals. This reward is so powerful that if allowed to, animals will administer brain stimulation at the expense of all other rewards, and they will eventually stop eating and die (Olds, 1956).

In the context of the assumption that reproductive success may be enhanced or, at least, not substantially impaired, it is possible to think of drug use in the evolutionary environment as being potentially adaptive.

For example, frequent chewing of coca leaves by some South Americans increases energy and vigor but does not apparently cause life-ruining (and presumably fitness-decreasing) addiction. It is possible that this gently, if artificially tweaked, positive mood could confer a social advantage to a coca chewer without serious consequences, except perhaps health problems in old age. If fitness gains from chewing were high, and costs were low, any psychological or physiological traits making coca chewing more likely could have been selected. In this theoretical case, increased coca-induced social success is traded for good health in old age, when most reproduction is probably already completed. The likelihood of this scenario actually having contributed to the evolution of 'addictability' is hard to gauge, and would depend upon the presence, and specific uses of psychoactive compounds in the evolutionary environment.

Constraints on the evolution of the brain might also be involved in why our brains are addiction-prone. The mesolimbic dopamine system appears to be a phylogenetically old brain structure. An analogous circuit is present in all mammals, reptiles, and even sea slugs. While it is possible that such a 'reward' circuit evolved independently multiple times due to convergent evolution, a more parsimonious explanation is that this is a conserved neural substrate mediating a basic aspect of psychology common to all these creatures. Our present understanding of the function of this system (guiding behavior toward or away from motivationally significant cues), fits the bill of such a basic psychological process. If mesolimbic dopamine system plays a fundamental, basic role in motivation, it is entirely possible that it is not very susceptible to modification by selective pressures that have occurred recently (pure drugs and methods of administration are new), and infrequently (most addicts recover before dying). In other words, a relatively weak selective pressure to limit addictability might not be sufficient to change greatly the functioning of a fundamental, well-integrated psychological process such as "wanting." Addiction was likely rare in the evolutionary environment, so a mechanism to shut off excessive "wanting" of inappropriate rewards might never have been selected for until very recently (Saah, 2005).

Today, in advanced civilizations, addiction, in its purist form, only leads to *"jails, institutions and death,"* to quote an old adage of Twelve Step recovery groups, such as Alcoholics Anonymous and Narcotics Anonymous. In modern society, the addict or alcoholic often has a responsibility for driving a car, holding a job, or providing for a family or significant other.

These responsibilities last long after reproductive age has come and gone. As stated earlier, the economic cost of drug and alcohol addiction on modern society is staggering. This includes costs related to crimes and incarceration, drug addiction treatment, medical costs from overdoses and drug related injuries and complications, time lost from work, and social welfare programs. Because drug addiction and alcoholism are diseases of the brain, which is the center of judgment and behavioral patterns, drug addicts and alcoholics have a disturbingly high propensity to commit unlawful and immoral acts to obtain these substances. Moreover, once under the influence of drugs and alcohol, the addict's inhibitions are drastically lowered with a sense of indestructibility, which leads to aggressive and irresponsible behavior. Nonetheless, it is estimated that every year over 60 percent of the human adult population experiments or routinely uses mood-altering substances 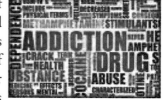 (NIDA, 2008). It seems that our motivation to alter our emotional state persists despite the risk of negative consequences or possible addiction.

John S.: Courage in a Bottle

John is good-looking young man, sixteen years old, and very interested in the opposite sex. He is "vertically impaired" (on the short size for his age) and down-right skinny. He has a wisp of facial hair under his nose. John wants a girl, but cannot get the courage to ask one out. At a party at a friend's house, the parents' liquor cabinet was raided and he had his first drink of hard liquor. When the booze hit his brain, the feeling was magic. He was relaxed and suddenly felt "tall and strong." He approached a cute young girl and struck up a conversation for the first time in his life. He found his courage in a bottle. He repeated this scenario many times until he finally got a date and a kiss. Later he found the same "courage" in marijuana and unknown small white pills he bought at school. His grades faltered, but he did not care. He found his answer to life in booze and other mood-altering drugs.

Chapter 3

Reward Centers of the Brain: Origins of Emotion, Memory, and Motivation

Admittedly, parts of this chapter explaining complex neuroanatomy with Latin nomenclature might be a bit onerous for some readers. I have made every attempt to simplify the terminology and make the information accessible without losing the message. *I must say, however, this is only the tip the iceberg of what we know today.* For example, every "part" I mention also has "subparts," and every connection I mention has a plethora of subconnections. This is all that we know, and we know very little, in my opinion.

The brain is an enormous data processor with an estimated 100 billion cells, and double-digit or quadruple-digit exponent of 100 billion connections between those cells. Replicating its most rudimentary capacities in the laboratory takes computers the size of refrigerators, even with today's byte storage and transmission technology. In 2010, Watson, a computer built by IBM to play Jeopardy on TV (remember Deep Blue, the chess player, 1997) and celebrate its 100th anniversary, has 15 terabytes of RAM and 2,880 processing cores. It plays a respectable round against a human, but it cannot nurse a baby or raise a family, and it is the size of ten refrigerators. And it makes mistakes. It is estimated by IBM techies that there are about fifteen petabytes of new data generated in the world news each day. *How many petabytes does it take to nurse a baby or raise a family? We know only a little.*

To those not particularly interested in neuroanatomy, I apologize. I think the salient points of this chapter can be gleaned by skimming the text and looking at the pictures, which is what I do when weary. I get weary of this stuff myself sometimes; but it is fascinating, absolutely Fascinating. *After all, essentially, it is what we are!*

The Limbic System

Buried within the depths of the brain are several large aggregates of neurons called "nuclei," which are preeminent in the control and mediation of memory, emotion, learning, dreaming, attention, and arousal, called the *limbic system.* The limbic system fundamentally determines our perception and expression of emotional, motivational, sexual, and social behavior, including the formation of loving attachments. *The limbic system is described as the background of emotional tone and is involved in monitoring, mediating and expressing motivational, sexual, and social behavior* (LeDoux, 1996, 2000). Indeed, the limbic system not only controls the capacity to experience love and sorrow, but it governs and monitors internal homeostasis (balance) and basic needs, such as hunger and thirst. *Given its exceedingly rudimentary function for survival of the organism, it harbors the fundamental reward centers of the brain* (Joseph, 1996). These reward centers are responsible for cravings for pleasure-inducing drugs (Childress, 1999).

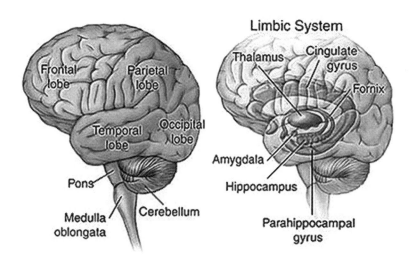

The limbic structures receive projections from all sensory receptors, which enable the individual to "judge" the appropriate response to sensory input. In sufficient intensity, any sensation (pressure, heat, sound, smell, movement, touch, etc.) will result in emotional characteristics leading to approach or avoidance. Fight or flight, attraction or avoidance, arousal or calming, hunger, thirst, satiation, fear, sadness, affection, happiness, and the control of aggression are all responses mediated by the limbic system (Joseph, 1996).

Although the neocortex is involved in rational thought and emotional expression, the subcortical limbic structures are the major sites for elicitation of emotional arousal (Joseph, 1996). The neocortical mantle surrounding the limbic system is associated with the conscious, rational mind. Sometimes, however, even in the most rational of humans, limbic-centered emotions can hijack the logical mind, the neocortex. Indeed, the old limbic brain is capable of completely overwhelming "the rational mind" due in part to the massive axonal projections (nerve branch connections) of the limbic system to the neocortex. *Emotions originating in the limbic system are a strong and potentially overwhelming force.* Although over the course of evolution a new brain (neocortex) has developed, *Homo sapiens* ("the wise man who knows he is wise") remains a creature of emotion.

Emotions can temporarily hijack, overwhelm, and snuff out the "rational mind." Because of our limbic roots, humans not uncommonly behave "irrationally" or in the "heat of passion," get into fights, and/or have sex with or scream and yell at strangers, thus acting enslaved to their immediate desires. We are known to fall "madly in love" and at other times, act in a blind rage, murdering another human being; sometimes that someone was "dear" to us.

The schism between the rational (neocortical) and the emotional (limbic) is real, and is due to the raw energy of emotion having its source in the nuclei of the ancient limbic system, which first made its appearance hundreds of millions of years before humans walked upon this earth and which continue to control and direct human behavior. The power of the limbic system cannot be ignored. Indeed, it is the power of the limbic system that is hijacked by substances of abuse.

Reward and Punishment: The Roots of Emotion

Emotion is conceptually rooted in the processing of reward and punishment (Rolls, 2000). Primary rewards satisfy intrinsic drives necessary for survival, and elicit positive emotional states. Areas of the limbic system are activated by primary rewards such as pleasant tastes, and by expectation of these rewards. Proxy awards—such as money, pictures of money, points score and tick marks—share similar reinforcing qualities in humans. Limbic structures and the perilimbic cortex are also activated by abstract rewards, such as the promise or depiction of money (Izuma, 2008). Activity in the orbitofrontal (inferior frontal) cortex and amygdala (small nucleus near the ear) is enhanced by pictures of foods, only when hungry, reflecting differences in reward perception and interpretation (Siep, 2009). Memory of these food stimuli is also greater when hungry and correlated with amygdala and orbitofrontal activity at the time of presentation.

When natural rewards or substances of abuse stimulate the brain reward pathway, there is a release of chemicals called neurotransmitters in synapses (gaps) between individual neurons. This release of neurotransmitters propagates a nerve impulse leading to subjective feelings of well-being (Koob, 1997). This brain reward system evolved to promote activities essential to species survival, such as sexual activity and feeding behaviors. Activities that activate this pathway become associated with "feeling good." Sexual intercourse causes release of chemicals in this pathway, as does eating chocolate. Thus, the reward pathway serves to promote survival of the species by rewarding behaviors necessary for continued survival: seeking food, reproduction, shelter, drink, etc.

Nuclei of the limbic system are involved in reward pathways for alcohol, opiates, and stimulants (Bardo, 1998). *Drugs of abuse stimulate this "brain reward" pathway generally in a greater fashion than good sex and good chocolate. This is because the active ingredient in addictive substances is concentrated though their manufacturing. This is why substance users experience a "high" when they use them.*

Core Reward Pathway

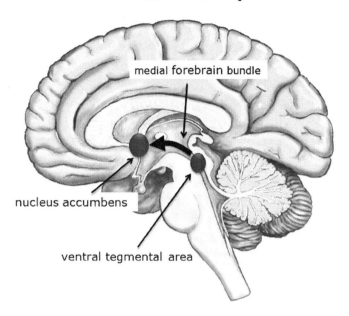

medial forebrain bundle

nucleus accumbens

ventral tegmental area

The reward pathway, located in the limbic system, is primarily made up of two core structures: the nucleus accumbens (NA) and the ventral tegmental area (VTA) connected by the medial forebrain bundle (MFB). The NA and the VTA are the most frequently implicated structures in the literature on drug reward (Lowinson, 1997). The MFB is composed of nerves that not only connect the VTA and NA to each other, but also connect these structures to other structures of the limbic system (Koob, 1997). In other words, the MFB is like a cable of neurons connecting the structures of the reward pathway with other brain structures. Experiments demonstrate that when this cable is cut, animals will decrease or stop self-administration of addictive drugs (Yeomans, 1982). Often the animals will also stop mating, eating and drinking; many die as a result. Thus, an intact MFB appears to be necessary for the brain-reward system to function properly.

Neurotransmitters of the Reward Pathway

Human motivational behavior is mediated primarily by dopaminergic (dopamine-containing) and serotonergic (serotonin-containing) neurotransmitter systems (LeDoux, 2000). The corticomesolimbic (cortex to limbic) dopaminergic system is the target of a wide range of drugs, including marijuana, alcohol and cocaine, increasing the transmission of dopamine in limbic nuclei (Koob, 1997). This system mediates emotion and controls reinforcement. Problematic use of drugs develops into addiction as the brain becomes dependent on the chemical neural homeostatic circuitry altered by the drug.

Dopamine

The primary neurotransmitter of the reward pathway is dopamine (Koob, 1997). Although drugs of abuse often act through separate mechanisms and on various locations in the brain reward system, they share a final common action in that they increase dopamine levels in the brain reward system. In general, drugs that are not abused have no effect on dopaminergic concentrations.

Other neurotransmitter systems of the brain are inextricably intertwined with the dopamine system. Thus, the neurotransmitter systems comprised of serotonin, endogenous opiates, as well as GABA also modulate dopamine levels in the brain reward pathway. Some mechanisms that may contribute to increasing dopamine levels include the blockade of re-uptake and stimulation of release.

Dopaminergic neurons form a neurotransmitter system that originates in brainstem nuclei (ventral tegmental area, or VTA) and hypothalamus. These project axons (branches) to larger areas of the brain which are typically divided into four major pathways (Ikemoto, 2007): (1) The *mesocortical pathway* connects the ventral tegmental area to the frontal lobe of the pre-frontal cortex. Neurons with somas (cell bodies) in the ventral tegmental area project axons (connections) into the pre-frontal cortex. (2) The *mesolimbic pathway* carries dopamine from the ventral tegmental area to the nucleus accumbens via the amygdala and hippocampus. The somas of the projecting neurons are in the ventral tegmental area. (3) The *nigrostriatal pathway* runs from the substantia nigra to the neostriatum. Neurons in the substantia nigra project axons into the caudate nucleus and putamen. The pathway is involved in the basal ganglia motor loop. (4) The *tuberoinfundibular pathway* runs from the hypothalamus to the pituitary gland. *This connection explains the effect of the dopamine-mediated reward pathway on hormones, like the stress hormones, cortisol. For instance, activation of the reward system, in most circumstances, causes decreases in the "stress" hormone, cortisol, and an increase in the ."comfort" hormone, oxytocin. Cortisol also is known to increase with heavy drug use and in withdrawal states.*

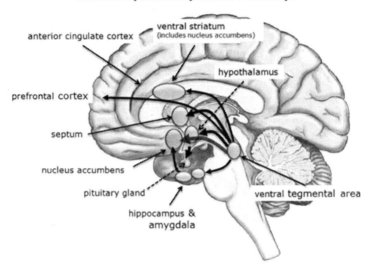

Reward System Dopamine Pathways

Normally, the dopaminergic neurons are only phasically active. When they are excited, they fire a barrage of action potentials (electrical impulses), and dopamine is released in the NA. The neurons of the NA are much more responsive to this increase in dopamine if there is coincident excitatory input from other structures such as the amygdala and orbitofrontal and prefrontal cortices. The activated NA neurons then project to the ventral striatum (back of the frontal lobes), where they inhibit the inhibitory GABA neurons. This inhibition in the striatum disinhibits the thalamic target of the limbic loop. The thalamus then innervates the cortical division of the limbic forebrain. This final connection is reinforced by activity in direct cortical projections from the dopaminergic neurons of the VTA. (You see, the connections get very complex, and this is only the tip of the iceberg—gives me a headache sometimes, too.)

Serotonin

Even though increased dopamine in the brain reward system is generally thought to be the final common pathway for the reinforcing properties of drugs, other neurotransmitters, such as serotonin, are involved in the modulation of both drug self-administration and dopamine levels (Bardo, 1998; Koob, 1997). Serotonin is stimulated by a small range of drugs and mediates arousal. Hallucinogens bind to serotonin receptors. Serotonin has been shown to help control wanting for ethanol and cocaine consumption (Saah, 2005). Serotonin may be important in modulating motivational factors, or the amount of work an individual is willing to perform to obtain a drug. Serotonergic neurons project both to the NA and VTA, and act to regulate dopamine release to the NA. However, the relationship between serotonin and dopamine release is complex in that serotonin has numerous receptor types and its regulation of dopamine release is at times inhibitory and at other times excitatory. Thus, serotonin modulates the reward pathway through various mechanisms by interacting with different receptors throughout the brain.

GABA

GABA (gamma-aminobutyric acid), another neurotransmitter involved in the modulation of dopaminergic reward systems, plays a role in the mediation of effects of many drugs of abuse (Olson, 2007). GABA is an inhibitory neurotransmitter located diffusely throughout the brain occurring in 30 to 40 percent of all synapses (second only to glutamate as a major brain neurotransmitter). It is most highly concentrated in the substantia nigra (brainstem nuclei) and globus pallidus nuclei of the basal ganglia (a.k.a. the striatum, back of the frontal lobe), followed by the hypothalamus (hormone center), the brainstem (breathing, heart rate, and reward centers), and the hippocampus (memory center).

Benzodiazepines enhance the effect of GABA, which results in sedative, hypnotic (sleep-inducing), anxiolytic (anti-anxiety), anticonvulsant, muscle relaxant and amnesic action. Ethanol also enhances the effects of GABA. The effects of benzodiazepines are often compared with those of alcohol.

Glutamate

Glutamate is the most common neurotransmitter in the brain. It is always excitatory, usually due to simple receptors that increase the flow of positive ions by opening ion-channels (Bardo, 1998). *Glutamate neurotransmitter systems do not produce feelings of reward; however, they connect reward centers with each other and the neocortex.* Glutamate binds to NMDA (*N*-methyl *D*-aspartate) synaptic receptors which are most densely concentrated in the cerebral cortex, hippocampus, amygdala, and basal ganglia. Increased alertness (or anxiety) due to caffeine may be due mainly to blockage of adenosine receptors that normally inhibit glutamate release.

The NMDA receptor is the only known receptor regulated both by a ligand (glutamate) and by voltage. NMDA receptors have a capacity for an activity-dependent increase in synaptic efficiency known as *"long-term potentiation"* (LTP) which is crucial to some forms of learning and memory. Inhibition of NMDA receptor activity (and LTP) is believed to be an important part of the way ethanol negatively affects brain learning and memory.

Reward System Glutamate Pathways

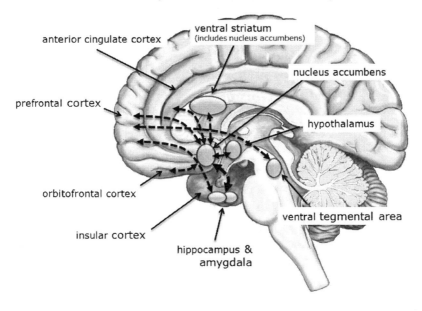

The Endogenous Opiates

Like dopamine, endogenous proteins called endorphins also motivate behavior (Koob, 1997). Although several endorphins have been identified, the two most prevalent are two pentapeptides named methionine (Met) enkephalin and leucine (Leu) enkephalin. Endorphins are partially responsible for the "high" one gets after vigorous exercise. Endorphin receptors, like dopamine receptors, have been discovered in vertebrates from the hagfish to man, suggesting that endorphin receptors also conferred a selective advantage to the organism (Joseph, 1996).

Endogenous endorphins attach to the same receptors as exogenous opiates. Through the same mechanism, they both increase dopamine in the brain reward pathway (Bozarth, 1987a-c, 1988). Opiates enhance dopamine-cell firing and increase metabolic indexes of dopamine release in the nucleus accumbens. Behavioral data also suggest that opiate administration activates the mesolimbic dopamine system; increased locomotor activity follows bilateral morphine injections into the ventral tegmental area (Smith, 1983). These studies provide neurochemical and behavioral data suggesting an enhancement of the mesolimbic dopamine system following opiate administration.

The highest levels of opiate receptors are found in areas of the limbic system and in the regions that have been implicated in the pathways involved in pain perception (Smith, 1983). To date, four opiate receptors have been cloned, the mu (μ) (MOP-R), kappa (κ) (KOP-R), delta (δ) (DOP-R), and NOP-R, the latter initially referred to as ORL-1 or nociceptin/orphanin FQ receptor. It is thought that the limbic system receptors may be involved in opiate-induced euphoria (or dysphoria) and in the affective aspects of pain perception.

All the endorphins, including the enkephalins, exhibit opiate-like activity (Bozarth, 1988). This activity includes analgesia, respiratory depression, and a variety of behavioral changes. The pharmacological effects of the enkephalins are very fleeting. The longer chain endorphins are more stable and produce long-lived effects. Thus, analgesia due to Y-endorphin (the most potent of all the endorphins so far found) can last three to four hours. All of the responses to endorphins are readily reversed by opiate antagonists, such as naloxone.

Integrated Structures of the Reward and Limbic Systems

The core structures of the brain reward pathway are located within and intimately connected to the limbic nuclei (LeDoux, 2000). The primary nuclei (or parts) of the limbic system include the hypothalamus, amygdala, hippocampus, sepal nuclei, and anterior cingulate gyrus. Also important in the function of the limbic system is the striatum, which includes the nucleus accumbens, ventral caudate nucleus, and putamen. The nucleus accumbens is an especially important structure of the brain reward pathway because drugs of abuse target it. Other structures important in brain reward include the amygdala and the ventral tegmental area (VTA). The perilimbic cortex and cortical areas surrounding the limbic system—including the cingulate gyrus (located above) and orbitofrontal cortex (located in front)—also are involved in the reward system. The prefrontal cortex, center of executive functioning, is the only extended cortical structure connected to the reward and limbic structures.

Limbic System

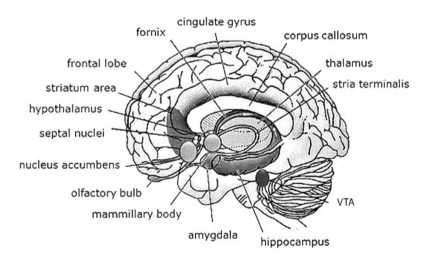

Using evidence from structural and functional magnetic resonance imaging (fMRI), researchers have identified multiple connections of the reward pathways. The central reward pathway of the brain (nucleus accumbens and ventral tegmental area) sends information to and receives input from many other brain structures: the reticular activating system (RAS) in the brainstem, limbic structures, the frontal cortex (executive control), the striatum (basal ganglia in back of frontal lobe), and the cerebellum.

Located in the brainstem, the RAS controls attention and arousal to various sensory inputs from our environment. It has diurnal activity and is responsible for us going to sleep. Limbic regions, such as the amygdala, the septum, and the thalamus, provide input to the reward pathway concerning motivational and emotional variables. Surrounding the amygdala is the insular cortex of the temporal lobe, also involved in emotional regulation and perception. Connections to the prefrontal cortex influence higher executive functions, such as judgment and decision-making. Other parts of the frontal lobe, the anterior cingulate cortex and the orbitofrontal cortex, are involved in emotional regulation and perception. The reward pathway also interacts with the basal ganglia (behind frontal lobe) and cerebellum (back base of the head) to modify motor activity.

Extended Reward and Oversight System

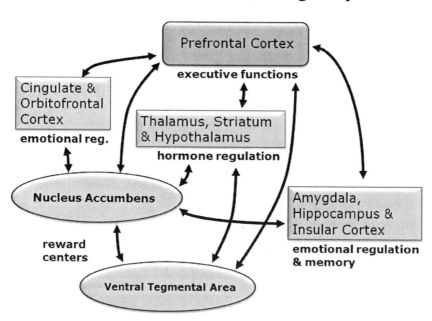

Using evidence from structural and functional magnetic resonance imaging (fMRI), researchers have proposed this model of brain regions involved in what they termed is the "extended reward and oversight system." (Adapted from Makris et al. 2008.)

In addition, the endocrine and the autonomic nervous systems interact with the reward system via the hypothalamus, an integral part of the limbic system, and the pituitary. These structures modulate the reward pathway and vice versa. The hypothalamus is involved in every aspect of endocrine, visceral, and autonomic functions, and it is able to influence eating, drinking, sexual activity, aversion, rage, and pleasure. Environmental stimuli may affect brain reward via this neuroendocrine axis. Given the connections with brain structures involved in higher cortical functions and the endocrine system, researchers have termed the sum of these connections the "extended reward and oversight system." (Makris, 2008) The intimate details of the interactions between the reward pathway and other regions of the brain are complex and beyond the scope of this text.

Role of Limbic Structures in the Formation of Emotions

There are two theories on the formation of emotions in the limbic system (Amaral, 2010). According to the James-Lange theory, developed at the turn of the century, the man perceives, let's say, a frightening animal and reacts with physical (neurovegetative) manifestations. As a consequence of such unpleasant physical reaction, he develops fear. Thus, in the James-Lange theory, emotion is reflexive in nature, bypassing higher cortical centers to lead directly to physical/visceral responses.

In 1929, Walter Cannon challenged James's theory and, with Phillip Bard, proposed the Cannon-Bard theory, which states that, when a person faces a stimulus or event, the nervous impulse travels straight to the thalamus, where the message is divided in two. One part of the message goes to the cortex to be interpreted as subjective experiences, such as fear, rage, sadness, joy, etc. The other part goes to the hypothalamus to determine the peripheral neurovegetative changes or symptoms associated with the emotion, such as dilated pupils, increased heart rate, or sweaty palms. According to the Cannon-Bard theory, physiological reactions and emotional experience occur simultaneously.

In 1937, the neurologist, James Papez, refined our understanding of the origin of emotion in the brain. Papez asserted that the experience of emotion was primarily determined by the cingulate cortex (inferior part of the frontal lobe) and, secondly, by other cortical areas, and emotional expression was thought to be governed by the hypothalamus (Papez, 1937). The cingulate gyrus projects to the hippocampus (memory), and the hippocampus projects to the hypothalamus (hormones) by way of the bundle of axons called the fornix. Hypothalamic impulses reach the cortex via relay in the anterior thalamic nuclei.

James Papez demonstrated that emotion is not a function of any specific brain center but of a circuit that involves four basic structures, interconnected through several nervous bundles: the hypothalamus with its mammallary bodies, the anterior thalamic nucleus, the cingulate gyrus and the hippocampus. This circuit (Papez circuit), acting in a harmonic fashion, is responsible for the central functions of emotion (affect), as well as for its peripheral expressions (symptoms).

More recently, Paul McLean, accepting the essential bases of the Papez proposal, created the *"denomination limbic system"* and added new structures to circuit: the orbitofrontal and orbitofrontal cortices, the parahippocampal gyrus, and important subcortical groupings, like the amygdala, the medial thalamic nucleus, the septal area, basal ganglia nuclei (ventral striatum), and a few brainstem formations (MacLean, 1952). It is important to stress that all these structures interconnect intensively, and none of them is *solely* responsible for any specific emotional state. However, some contribute more than others for a specific kind of emotion.

We will see in the following chapters that these brain structures are activated in cravings and can be strengthened through meditation. For the sake of completeness, I will review, one by one, the best-known structures of the limbic system and their functions. (If you're weary of this stuff, please, just look at the pictures and move on.)

Hypothalamus

The hypothalamus could be considered *the most "primitive" aspect of the limbic system* (LeDoux, 1996). Although primitive, the functioning of this sexually dimorphic structure is exceedingly complex. The hypothalamus regulates internal homeostasis (balanced states, such as electrolytes, metabolism, and body temperature), including the experience of hunger and thirst, which can trigger rudimentary sexual behaviors or generate feelings of extreme rage or pleasure. In conjunction with the pituitary, the hypothalamus is a major manufacturer/secretor of hormones and hormone-release factors (triggers), including those involved in the stress response and feelings of depression. The hypothalamus governs the pituitary gland forming what is known as the hypothalamic-pituitary axis. *Through the hypothalamic-pituitary axis, our emotions influence our hormonal states.*

The hypothalamus has been found to play a central role in the formation of emotion (LeDoux, 2000). Specifically, its lateral (outside) parts seem to be involved with pleasure and rage, while the medial (inside) part is likely to be involved with aversion, displeasure, and a tendency for uncontrollable and loud laughing. However, in general terms, *the hypothalamus has more to do with the expression (symptomatic manifestations) of emotions than with the genesis of the affective states.* When the physical symptoms of emotion appear, the threat they pose returns, via hypothalamus, to the limbic centers and, thence, to the pre-frontal cortex, increasing anxiety. This negative feedback mechanism can be so strong as to generate an emotional state of panic, or extreme physiological state of the "panic attack."

Additionally, there are many complex behaviors that are patterned by the hypothalamus, including sexual responses. The preoptic area of the hypothalamus is one of the areas of greatest sexual dimorphism (i.e., difference in structure between the sexes) and, along with the septal nuclei, is an area of gonadotropin-releasing hormone projections to the median eminence region of the hypothalamus. These sexual responses involve autonomic, endocrine, and behavioral responses.

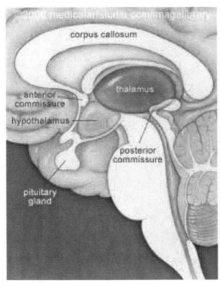 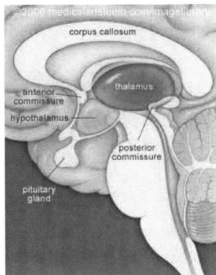

Thalamus

The thalamus is the relay center for emotional reactions. Stimulation of the medial dorsal (inside and posterior) and anterior nuclei of the thalamus is associated with changes in emotional reactivity. However, the importance of these nuclei on the regulation of emotional behaviors is not due to the thalamus itself, but to the connections of these nuclei with other limbic system structures. The medial dorsal nucleus makes connections with cortical zones of the pre-frontal cortex and with the hypothalamus. The anterior nuclei connect with the mammallary bodies (brainstem), and through them, via the fornix, with the hippocampus and the cingulate gyrus, thus taking part in the Papez circuit.

Amygdala

The amygdala has been dubbed the "fear center." It is a small almond-shaped structure, deep inside the antero-inferior region of the temporal lobe (in front of the ear), which connects with the hippocampus, the septal nuclei, the prefrontal area, and the medial dorsal nucleus of the hypothalamus. These connections make it possible for the amygdala to play its important role on the mediation and control of major emotional states. *The amygdala, being the center for identification of danger, is fundamental for self-preservation. When triggered, it gives rise to fear and anxiety, which lead the animal into a stage of alertness, getting ready to "fight or flight."* Experimental destruction of both amygdalae (there are two of them, one in each hemisphere) tames the animal, which becomes sexually non-discriminative, unaffectionate and indifferent to danger (Amaral, 2003). The electrical stimulus of these structures elicits crises of violent aggression (Davis, 2001). Humans with marked lesions of the amygdala, loose the affective meaning of the perception of outside information, like the sight of a well-known person. It contains neurons that become activated in response to the human face and become activated in response to the direction of someone else's gaze (Zald, 2003). The subject knows exactly who the person is but is not capable of deciding whether he likes or dislikes him (or her). The amygdala is implicated in the seeking of loving attachments and the formation of long-term emotional memories.

Therefore, the role of the amygdala in memory and learning seems to involve activities related to reward, orientation, and attention, as well as emotional arousal and social-emotional recognition (Rolls, 2000). *The amygdala is immediately adjacent to and richly connected with the hippocampus, the center of memory formation.* If some event is associated with substantive positive or negative emotional states it is more likely to be learned and remembered. That is, reward increases the probability of attention being paid to a particular stimulus or consequence as a function of its association with reinforcement (Zald, 2003).

Moreover, the amygdala appears to reinforce and maintain hippocampal activity via the identification of motivationally significant information and the generation of pleasurable rewards (through action on the lateral hypothalamus). However, the amygdala and hippocampus act differentially in regard to the effects of positive versus negative reinforcement on learning and memory, particularly when highly stressed or repetitively aroused in a negative fashion. For example, whereas the hippocampus is activated in response to noxious stimuli, the amygdala increases its activity following the reception of rewarding or aversive stimuli (Davis, 2001).

In this regard, it appears that the amygdala is responsible for emotional memory formation, whereas the hippocampus is responsible for storing verbal, visual, spatial, and contextual details in memory. Thus, in rats and primates, damage to the hippocampus can impair retention of context and contextual fear conditioning, but it has no effect on the retention of the fear itself or the fear reaction to the original cue (Amaral 1992, 2003; LeDoux 1992, 1996). In these instances, fear-memory is retained due to preservation of the amygdala.

Hippocampus

The hippocampus is the center of new memory formation. The hippocampus is unique in that, unlike the amygdala and other structures, almost all of its input from the neocortex is relayed via the cortex surrounding it, called the entorhinal cortex (LeDoux, 1996). The hippocampus is exceedingly important in memory, acting to place various short-term memories into long-term storage. Presumably, the hippocampus encodes new information during the storage and consolidation (long-term storage) phase and assists in the gating of afferent streams of information destined for the neocortex by filtering or suppressing irrelevant sense data that may interfere with memory consolidation. Moreover, it is believed that via the process of *long-term potentiation* (the accentuation of synaptic activity between neurons), the hippocampus is able to track information as it is stored in the neocortex and to form conjunctions between synapses and different brain regions that process and store associated memories. The hippocampus has several other functions. It helps control corticosteroid production. It also has significant contribution to understanding spatial relations within the environment and declarative memory (Davidson, 2000).

There are several types of memory (Joseph, 1996): *Explicit* or declarative memory refers to the memory of facts and events. Any memory that can be completely explained in words is of this type. *Implicit* or non-declarative memory, however, is also very important. The learning of skills, as well as associative learning, such as conditioned and emotional responses, are common examples of non-declarative or implicit memory. Explicit memory depends on the medial temporal lobe and the relationship between the hippocampus and entorhinal region of the parahippocampal gyrus.

There are several areas involved in explicit memory. The hippocampus plays a critical role in short-term memory, which is absolutely necessary if long-term memory patterns are to be established. *Lesions of the hippocampus do not affect old, established memories. These lesions affect new declarative learning.* Ultimately, memory storage is transferred to other areas of the cerebral cortex, and the location of encoding of these memories may be a function of the type of memory. Established memories involve association areas in the frontal lobe and parietal-temporal-occipital association cortex. The hippocampus is not only active in encoding memories but also in retrieving them. Activation of the hippocampus can be seen in this case of learning about new surroundings and retrieving directions. *When both hippocampi (right and left) are destroyed, nothing new can be retained in the memory.* The subject quickly forgets any recently received messages. The intact hippocampus allows the animal to compare the conditions of a present threat with similar past experiences, thus enabling it to choose the best option, in order to guarantee its own survival.

Septal Nuclei

The septal nuclei are within the septum (the terms are interchangeable) and are interconnected with the hippocampus, as well as the hypothalamus and amygdala (Joseph, 1996). The septal nuclei appear to function in an inhibitory manner, dampening and quieting arousal and limbic system functioning. As such, they reduce extremes of emotionality and maintain the individual in a state of quiet readiness to respond. In contrast to the amygdala which promotes social behavior, the septum counters socializing tendencies. The septal nuclei also are interconnected with and share a counterbalancing relationship with the amygdala, particularly in regard to hypothalamic activity and emotional and sexual arousal. For example, whereas the amygdala promotes indiscriminate contact seeking, and perhaps promiscuous sexual activity, the septal nuclei inhibits these tendencies, thus assisting in the formation of selective and more enduring emotional attachments. *The septum has been associated with different kinds of pleasant sensations, mainly those related to sexual experiences. Centers for orgasm—four for women and one for men—are found in the septum (not fair).*

Nucleus Accumbens

The nucleus accumbens (NA) is a collection of neurons within the posterior and inferior part of the frontal lobe called the *striatum* (Wu, 2010). The NA and the olfactory tubercle (nerves from the nose) collectively form the ventral striatum, which is part of the basal ganglia. It is located where the head of the caudate and the anterior portion of the putamen meet just lateral to the septum pellucidum.

The NA is thought to play a central role in reward and pleasure. Dopaminergic input from the ventral tegmental area is thought to modulate the activity of neurons within the nucleus accumbens. In 1956, James Olds implanted electrodes into the NA of the rat and found that the rat chose to press a lever that stimulated it (Olds, 1956). It continued to prefer this over eating or drinking, even to the point of starvation. This suggests that the area is the *pleasure center* of the brain. These terminals are also the site of action of addictive drugs, which cause a many-fold increase in dopamine levels in the nucleus accumbens. *Almost every recreational drug has been shown to increase dopamine levels in the nucleus accumbens.*

Although the NA has traditionally been studied for its role in addiction, it plays an equal role in processing many rewards, such as food and sex. A recent study found that it is involved in the regulation of emotions induced by pleasant music, perhaps consequent to its role in mediating dopamine release (Menon, 2005). Many people who, for a genetic error, have a reduction of D2 (dopamine) receptors in the accumbens nucleus, become, sooner or later, incapable of obtaining gratification from the common pleasures of life (Lu, 1998). Thus, they seek atypical and noxious "pleasurable" alternatives, like alcoholism, cocaine addiction, impulsive gambling, and compulsion for sweet foods. The NA has been targeted by stereotactic surgery for ablation as a treatment in China for alcoholism (Wu, 2010).

The NA has rich connections with multiple brain structures: The output neurons of the nucleus accumbens send axon projections to the ventral analog of the globus pallidus—known as the ventral pallidum (VP) which is part of the striatum—which is deep to the frontal lobe. The VP, in turn, projects to the medial dorsal nucleus of the dorsal thalamus, which projects to the prefrontal cortex. Other output neurons from the nucleus accumbens include connections with the substantia nigra and the pontine reticular formation (in the brainstem). Major inputs to the nucleus accumbens include prefrontal association cortices, amygdala, and dopaminergic neurons located in the ventral tegmental area (VTA), which connect via the mesolimbic pathway. Thus, the nucleus accumbens is often described as one part of a mesocorticolimbic loop. The septal nuclei are not directly connected to the nucleus accumbens, however.

Ventral Tegmental Area

The ventral tegmentum (*tegmentum* is Latin for "covering"), better known as the *ventral tegmental area* (VTA), is a group of neurons located close to the midline on the floor of the midbrain. *The VTA is the origin of the dopaminergic cell bodies of the mesocorticolimbic dopamine system and is widely implicated in the drug and natural reward circuitry of the brain.* It is important in cognition, motivation, drug addiction, and several psychiatric disorders. The VTA contains neurons that project to numerous areas of the brain, from the prefrontal cortex to the brainstem and everywhere in between.

The VTA has also been shown to process various types of emotional output from the amygdala, where it may also play a role in avoidance and fear conditioning. Electrophysiological recordings have demonstrated that VTA neurons respond to novel stimuli, unexpected rewards, and reward-predictive sensory cues (Margolis, 2006).

The two primary efferent (output) fiber projections of the VTA are the mesocortical and the mesolimbic pathways. Three less important pathways also exist: the mesostriatal, the mesodiencephalic, and the mesorhombencephalic pathways.

The large mesolimbic pathway projects primarily to the NA and the olfactory tubercle via the medial forebrain bundle. The projection is so named to contrast it with the nigro-striatal dopamine system that runs parallel to it but connects the substantia nigra to the dorsal striatum. Other projections of the VTA dopamine neurons include the limbic-related regions (i.e. septum, hippocampus, amygdala, and prefrontal cortex). The mesocortical pathway projects to sensory, motor, limbic, and polysensory association cortices. The prefrontal, orbitofrontal, and cingulate cortices receive the majority of innervation from the VTA.

Almost all areas receiving projections from the VTA project back to it as afferent (input) projections (Oades, 1987). Thus, the *VTA* is reciprocally connected with a wide range of structures throughout the brain suggesting that it has a role in the control of function in the phylogenetically new and highly developed neocortex, as well as that of the phylogenetically older limbic areas.

There are excitatory glutaminergic input neurons that arise from almost every structure that project into the VTA, except the NA and the lateral septum (Wu, 1996). These glutaminergic input neurons play a key role in regulating VTA cell firing. When the glutaminergic neurons are activated, the firing rates of the dopamine neurons increase in the VTA and induce burst firing. *Studies have shown that these glutaminergic actions in the VTA are critical to the effects of drugs of abuse.*

Other input neurons into the VTA are mainly GABAergic and, thus, inhibitory. There is a substantial pathway from the subpallidal GABAergic area to the VTA (Olson, 2007). When this pathway is activated, there is an increase in the dopamine release in the mesolimbic pathway, which amplifies locomotor activity.

The *"limbic loop"* is loop of connections among the VTA, limbic structures, ventral pallidum, thalamus, and frontal cortex. The midbrain VTA projects neuromodulatory dopamine neurons to the ventral pallidum; the ventral pallidum makes internuclear connections to the thalamus, which projects to the cortex, thus completing the loop. The limbic loop, therefore, represents connections between subcortical and cortical structures. Most of the neuronal formations involved belong to the limbic system. This is the reason the cortical structures of the limbic loop represent our top executive level, which decides what we do and what we will not do in order to comply with motivational stimuli and contexts. *By means of the limbic loop the unconsciously working limbic centers shape our conscious experiences as to feelings (positive or negative), motivational goals and the intensity of our desire to bring them to reality.*

Prefrontal Cortex

The prefrontal cortex is in the front of the brain, behind the forehead. The orbitofrontal cortex is the portion of the frontal lobe over the orbits. *Both the prefrontal and orbitofrontal cortices are extremely well developed in humans and are critical to judgment, insight, motivation and mood.* It is also important for conditioned emotional reactions. The prefrontal cortex receives input from other areas of the limbic cortex, from the amygdala and from septal nuclei, and has reciprocal connections with each of these areas and with the thalamus. The frontal lobe underwent a great deal of development during the evolution of mammals. It is especially large in man and in some species of dolphins. *The frontal cortex does not belong to the traditional limbic circuit, but its intense bi-directional connections with limbic structures account for the important role it plays in the genesis, expression and modulation of emotional states.*

When the pre-frontal cortex suffers a lesion, the subject loses his sense of social responsibility as well as the capacity for concentration and abstraction. In some cases, although consciousness and some cognitive functions, like speech, remain intact, the subject can no longer solve problems, even the most elementary ones. When pre-frontal lobotomy was used for treatment of certain psychiatric disturbances, the patients entered into a stage of "affective buffer," no longer showing any sign of joy, sadness, hope or despair. In their words or attitudes, no traces of affection could be detected (Davidson, 2000). Damage to the prefrontal area produces difficulties with abstract reasoning, judgment, moods, and puzzle solving. The effect of frontal lobe damage on mood depends on the specific part of the prefrontal cortex damaged. The patient's behavior is often described as tactless. Also, this part of the cortex can be strongly affected by alcohol and drugs of abuse (more in Chapter 6). Similarly, lesions of the orbitofrontal cortex lead to decreased emotional reactivity and antisocial behavior (Damasio, 1994).

As previously described, there are pathways through the prefrontal cortex that are involved in reinforcement of behaviors and in "reward"

(Lammel, 2008). Electrical stimulation of these sites is highly reinforcing for behavior. Many of these pathways involve dopamine and are commonly affected by addictive drugs. Habituation in these pathways with chronic administration of addicting drugs is one of the most important targets of addiction research.

Various addictive compounds affect activity of the dopamine transmission in the nucleus accumbens (mesolimbic) and frontal cortical (mesocortical) systems (Koob, 1997). Additionally, these pathways appear to be functionally unbalanced in patients with schizophrenia. It appears that patients with schizophrenia have diminished dopamine effects through mesocortical systems to the prefrontal cortex (Lieberman, 1987). This could produce symptoms, such as social withdrawal and diminished emotional responsiveness. Concurrently, there is a relative increase in dopamine effects via the mesolimbic system to the ventral striatal system, resulting in positive symptoms of delusions and hallucinations.

Cingulate Gyrus

The cingulate gyrus (or cortex) is a deep part of the frontal lobe located in the medial (inside) side of the brain immediately above the corpus callosum (principal fiber bundle connecting the two cerebral hemispheres). There is still much to be learned about this gyrus, but it is already known that its frontal part coordinates smells and sights with pleasant memories of previous emotions. *The cingulate gyrus appears to have a primary role in attention and focus.* This region also participates in the emotional reaction to pain and in the regulation of aggressive behavior. Wild animals, submitted to the ablation of the cingulate gyrus (cingulectomy), become totally tamed. The cutting of a single bundle of this gyrus (cingulotomy) reduces pre-existing depression and anxiety levels, by interrupting neural communication across the Papez circuit (Bush, 2000).

The anterior cingulate cortex (ACC) is considered a transitional cortex or mesocortex and, as such, is part of the perilimbic cortex surrounding and connected to limbic nuclei (Bush, 2000). *The ACC is intimately interconnected with the hypothalamus, amygdala, septal nuclei, and hippocampus, and participates in memory and emotion including the experience of pain, misery, and anxiety, and is directly implicated in the evolution and expression of maternal behavior.* It is also the most "vocal" aspect of the brain, active during language tasks, and generates emotional-melodic aspects of speech which is expressed via interconnections with the right and left frontal speech areas. Thus, the ACC is implicated in the more-cognitive aspects of social-emotional behavior, including language and the establishment of long-term attachments beginning with the mother-infant bond.

The ACC is broadly described as belonging to the *"limbic lobe,"* given its expensive connections to subcortical structures such as the amygdala (Rolls, 2000). Several investigators have suggested a functional segregation, whereby the more-dorsal, posterior division is involved in cognitive tasks while the more ventral, anterior portion serves emotional functions (Bush, 2000). Lesions to the ACC result in a variety of emotional disturbances, including apathy and emotional instability. *The ACC is involved in a form of attention that serves to regulate both cognitive and emotional processing, and is closely interconnected to the prefrontal cortex.*

Therefore, the ACC interacts with the prefrontal cortex to regulate tasks with cognitive and affective components during an emotional response. More generally, the ACC is posited to be involved in the assessment of salience in motivational and emotional information and the regulation of emotional responses. The ACC has also been linked to the mediation of emotional arousal, and its activity appears to be more pronounced when external information requires additional processing with conflicting internal states. *Thus, activity in the ACC correlates with emotional awareness to both perceived and recall-generated emotion, suggesting its role in detecting emotional salience* (Bush, 2000).

Ventral Striatum

The *ventral striatum* (VS) refers to the front part of the corpus striatum, located deep to the frontal lobe. The VS includes several structures including the nucleus accumbens, olfactory tubercle and frontal parts of the caudate nucleus and putamen. The most important part of the ventral striatum, for the purpose of this discussion, is the nucleus accumbens (located at the bottom of the VS), which is an important target of dopaminergic projections from the ventral tegmental area.

Neuroimaging Studies of Reward and Emotion

As stated earlier, emotion is conceptually rooted in the processing of reward and punishment. Primary rewards satisfy intrinsic drives necessary for survival, and elicit positive emotional states. Imaging studies using functional magnetic resonance imaging (fMRI) have shown that brain areas including the orbitofrontal cortex and ventral striatum are activated by primary rewards, such as pleasant tastes, and by expectation of these rewards (Phan, 2004), but these areas are also activated by abstract rewards, such as the promise or depiction of money (Izuma, 2008). Activity in the orbitofrontal cortex (and amygdala) is enhanced by pictures of foods, but only when hungry (Siep, 2008), reflecting the differences in perception of the potential salience of the reward. Memory of these food stimuli is also greater when hungry and correlates with amygdala and orbitofrontal activity at the time of presentation. These imaging studies provide strong evidence for participation of the human orbitofrontal cortex and ventral striatum in immediate, prospective, and mnemonic processing of rewards.

Brain Regions Activated by Emotions

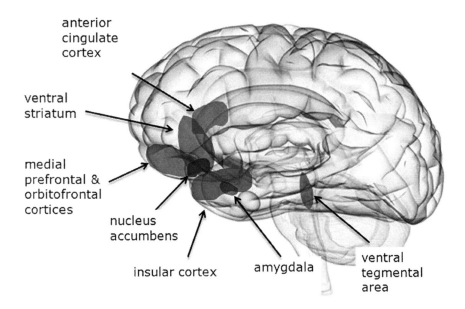

The foremost brain region implicated in emotion is the amygdala, positioned within the medial portion of the temporal lobe. Based on both animal work, human lesion, and imaging studies, the amygdala has been consistently implicated in fear conditioning (Amaral, 1992, 2003). In imaging studies, it is consistently activated when the subject is shown fearful facial expressions and reports feelings of fear (Hariri, 2002). Neuroscientists have found that the amygdalar response to fearful faces showed a significant interaction with the intensity of emotion, increasing with increasing fearfulness (Morris, 1998, 1999). Hence, the amygdalar activations may serve to signal threat, rather than evoke emotions of fear, and may serve a more general function to alert the organism toward salient cues. For example, the amygdala has been shown to govern judgments about the extent of trustworthiness as judged from facial expressions (Hamman, 2002).

However, other studies have shown that activation of the amygdala may not be entirely specific to fear-related or negative emotions. For example, amygdalar activations occur to various positive or pleasant stimuli, such as happy faces (Wright, 2002). Several studies have reported amygdalar responses to both appetitive (positive) and aversive (negative) stimuli (Zald, 2003). *Thus, the amygdala may not exclusively respond to particular positive or negative stimuli, but may respond more generally to salient characteristics of emotional stimuli and their potential for producing a substantive positive or negative emotional response.*

As remarked earlier, the anterior cingulate cortex (ACC) is posited to be involved in the assessment of salience in motivational and emotional information and the regulation of emotional responses. The ACC has also been linked to the mediation of emotional arousal and its activity appears to be more pronounced when external information requires additional processing with conflicting internal states (Critchley, 2000b, 2001, 2002). Furthermore, activity in the ACC during functional MRI exams has been shown to correlate with emotional awareness to both film and recall-generated emotion, suggesting its role in detecting emotional signals from both exteroceptive and interoceptive cues (Lane, 1997a-c). Lane and colleagues (1997a) also reported that the ACC activated when subjects attended to their internal, emotional state, but not when they attended to external, non-affective characteristics of a picture stimulus, such as deciding whether a scene was indoors or outdoors.

As a detector of salient information in general, the ACC could serve to allocate brain resources, heighten sensitivity, and direct attention to environmental cues produced by the evocative stimulus (Lane, 1997a-c). The specific emotion, sadness, was particularly associated with a region within the ACC, namely the subcallosal cingulate cortex (SCC). Approximately 46 percent of sadness induction studies reported activation of the ventral/subgenual ACC, over twice as frequently as any other specific emotion. Interestingly, alterations in SCC activity have been found in resting-state studies of patients with clinical depression, a mood disorder characterized by sustained sadness (Liotti, 2001). Specifically within smaller areas of the ACC (subgenual portion), physiological activity appears to be elevated during the depressed phase of some major depressive disorder subtypes (Drevets, 1998; Liotti, 2001). Activity in the subgenual cingulate appears to normalize when depressed subjects respond to pharmacologic treatment (Liotti, 2001).

Tasks inducing emotions in subjects often do so by having them evoke memories or imagery of personally relevant affectively laden autobiographical life events that require explicit, intensive, cognitive effort. Accordingly, the recollection/recall induction of emotion specifically activated the anterior cingulate; 50 percent of recall induction studies reported ACC activations, versus 31 percent and 0 percent of visual and auditory-based emotion studies, respectively (Liotti, 2001). *Cognitive tasks often engage the ACC and, therefore, this association suggests that recalled emotions involve cognitive activity,* as noted by several laboratories (Reiman, 1997). Given its known cognitive functions—including modulation of attention and executive functions, and interconnections with subcortical limbic structures—the ACC's involvement in cognitive induction of emotional response is not surprising. A small area at the top front of the ACC activated more during functional MRI exams when subjects imagined positive rather than negative future events (Lane, 1999). Activation was especially strong in subjects who scored high on scales of optimism. The researchers propose that this portion of the anterior cingulate cortex weighs emotional, motivational and autobiographical information with an eye for the positive.

The insular cortex within the temporal lobe has been shown to be consistently activated in emotive paradigms. This area surrounds the amygdala and hippocampus. Functional MRI studies of emotional recall reported activation of the temporal lobe insula compared with other emotion induction paradigms. Imaging studies have specifically found that emotional recall, but not emotional film viewing, engaged the insula. These findings as well as earlier studies on non-human primates support the notion that the insula is preferentially involved in the evaluative, experiential, or expressive aspects of "internally generated" emotions (Reiman, 1997)

Anatomically, the insula shares connections with the amygdala. Through these pathways, the insula relays interoceptive information to the amygdala and can communicate information based on internal somatic sensations evoked by emotional stimuli (Craig, 2002). Studies have observed that the insula responds more generally to aversive or threat-related processing, including not only disgust but also fear (Schienle, 2002). Animal studies have demonstrated that the insula is important for conditioned aversive responses, and recent human imaging studies link it the perception and experience of pain and anticipatory anxiety and other general negative emotional states, such as guilt (Shin, 2000). These findings point to the role of the insula as mediating responses to aversive or withdrawal-inducing stimuli.

Phan (2004) found that 60 percent of imaging studies on emotional recall reported activation of the insula compared with other emotion induction paradigms. Lane and colleagues (1997) and Reiman and colleagues (1997) specifically found that emotional recall, but not emotional film viewing, engaged the insula. These findings as well as earlier studies on non-human primates (Augustine, 1996) support the notion that the insular cortex is preferentially involved in the evaluative, experiential, or expressive aspects of "internally generated" emotions.

The insula seems to integrate emotionally relevant information between somatic internal feelings with external cues (Damasio, 1999). Such a process is evolutionarily adaptive in the service of providing a basis for implicit awareness of the physical self across time. Researchers have proposed that the insula may participate in the evaluation of the "interoceptive emotional significance" as an alarm center for internally sensed dangers or homeostatic changes (Reiman, 1997). Such an "internal alarm" hypothesis is consistent with the findings that insular activity is increased in response to all aversive stimuli that evoke visceral/somatic sensations. These involuntary "gut feelings" guide behavioral decisions by assigning emotional significance to a particular stimulus being experienced.

In addition to the cingulate gyrus and insula, the perilimbic medial prefrontal cortex (MPFC) is consistently activated in imaging studies in response to emotional stimuli, and its activation is not specific to a specific emotion (Phan, 2004). While there may not be a particular brain region that is absolutely necessary for all emotional functions, the common activation of the MPFC may reflect aspects shared across different emotional tasks. *These findings suggest that the MPFC may have a "general" role in emotional processing* (e.g., appraisal/evaluation, experience, response) (Lane, 1997a, 1997b). Emotional films, pictures, and recall as wells as positive and negative emotion, happiness, sadness, disgust, and the mixture of these emotions all separately engaged the MPFC. One possibility, therefore, is that the MPFC may be involved in the cognitive aspects (e.g., attention to emotion, appraisal/identification of emotion, awareness of emotion) that are closely intertwined with emotional processing (Drevets, 1998).

Functional MRI of Monetary Reward

nucleus accumbens

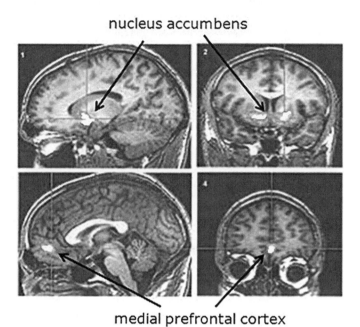

medial prefrontal cortex

Functional MRI of person experiencing a reward and happiness showing activity in the nucleus accumbens, anterior cingulate cortex nucleus accumbens and medial prefrontal cortex (from Peterson, 2005, with permission)

Activation of the MPFC could also involve the regulation of emotional states. The MPFC—with extensive connections to subcortical limbic structures including the amygdala—constitutes a "perilimbic" cortex, an interaction zone between emotive and cognitive processing (Lane, 1997c). *Given its connections to subcortical limbic structures, the MPFC could serve as a modulator of intense emotional responses, especially those generated by the amygdala.* Several lines of evidence support such an interpretation (Phan, 2004). PET (positron emission tomography) studies of glucose metabolism in the MPFC have shown that glucose metabolism in the MPFC inversely correlates with glucose metabolism of the amygdala (Abercromie, 1998). Similar studies have shown that activity in the amygdaloid region is attenuated while the MPFC and cingulate sulcus are activated during a cognitive appraisal condition of aversive visual stimuli (versus passive viewing) and that activity in MPFC is inversely related to that within the amygdala during emotional experience (Taylor, 2003). Recent studies that examine brain activation from cognitive reappraisal (an emotion regulation strategy) and cognitive volitional inhibition of emotionally evocative stimuli have observed engagement of the MPFC (Hariri, 2003). Deactivation of the amygdala has been observed in several tasks that involve higher cognitive processing and MPFC activity (Drevets, 1998). If responses in the amygdala to emotional evocation can be modulated by cognitive tasks, the MPFC appears to be the main anatomic structure that modulates this limbic activity.

The James-Lange model of emotional processing is that of a reflex: an "exciting" stimulus automatically elicits a motor or autonomic response (Wager, 2003). The automatic unconscious elicitation of emotion has been examined using functional imaging using subliminal presentation of face-stimuli. When an image of a face is shown very briefly (less than 300 milliseconds) it is registered in the visual cortex, but not in the higher cognitive centers; it is essentially "unseen." An unseen face represents a potential threat; therefore, the stimulus still evokes amygdalar activation (and a bodily arousal response) but no ACC or MPFC activity (Morris, 1998, 1999; Critchley, 2002). A subcortical route is implicated in mediating this unconscious processing of emotional stimulus, bypassing temporal and frontal cortices associated with conscious awareness and detailed feature processing of the stimuli (Wright, 2002; Rotshtein, 2001). Since survival is often dependent on a rapid response, a fast (subcortical) pathway evokes alertness and escape behavior to minimally processed, potentially threatening stimuli.

A second pathway via cortex, according to the Cannon-Baird and Papez theories, provides for a more detailed representation of the potential threat, enabling correction or reinforcement of the immediate fear response. Complex environmental and social stimuli may evoke emotions by virtue of their direct or implicit motivational meanings. Facial cues, such as an eye-gaze, beauty, and more elusive judgments of social potential, also share the motivational properties of primary reinforcers. The perception of attractive faces is associated with enhanced activity in "reward centers," such as ventral striatum, which is maximal when an eye gaze is directed at the viewer (Winston, 2002). "Romantic love" as expressed in the face of a loved one evokes a pattern of striatal, cingular and insular activity (Bartels, 2000).

Complex visual scenes and individual words may be rated according to emotive power or emotional content. A set of pictures, the International Affective Picture System (IAPS), comprises a large range of scenes that vary in their emotional valence (positive and negative) and their evocation of subjective arousal. In a combined fMRI (functional MRI) and MEG (magneto-encephalography) study, negative pictures activated the medial orbitofrontal cortex, whereas positive pictures preferentially activated the lateral orbitofrontal cortex (Northoff, 2000). The MEG data indicated a more rapid processing of emotional pictures, particularly those with negative content, than non-emotional pictures. Amygdala responses are reportedly enhanced by emotional words and positive emotional words that also activate reward-related regions of the ventral striatum (Hamman, 2002). In contrast, perception of humor is reported to activate medial prefrontal cortex (Phan, 2004).

The role of *bodily arousal states* has been emphasized in many theories of emotion (LeDoux, 1996, 2000). Neuroimaging studies have shown that brain regions implicated in emotional processing are involved at some level in control of autonomic responses and peripheral arousal states. *These studies implicate anterior cingulate, medial prefrontal, and insula cortices in generation and representation states of autonomic arousal.* In perhaps what may be considered the most interesting neuroimaging experiment of emotion, a recent functional MRI study used a direct measure of sexual arousal as a stimulus when male subjects watched pornography or sport films. Regional activity within the insula, basal ganglia, and cingulate cortex, as well as visual and somatosensory cortices, correlated positively with sexual arousal (Park, 2001). It is noteworthy that much less activity was attributable to the stimuli themselves compared with activity directly correlated with physiological changes (i.e. penile turgidity).

Summary

The use and abuse of mood-altering drugs are often conceptualized within the framework of reinforcement-related behaviors and attempts at modulation of emotion. Those who use mood-altering substances do so to either mitigate negative emotional states or accentuate positive ones. Neuroimaging, laboratory, and clinical studies of the limbic system and related structures continue to provide insights into the functional contributions of discrete brain regions to the development of addiction.

Knowledge of the anatomical and functional basis of emotion gives us the opportunity to understand the effect of mood-altering substances on the brain's reward and emotive centers. *These studies afford us a basis to ascertain the effect of recovery programs on reclaiming these centers, via endogenous cognitive and spiritual practices, from the grips of exogenous drugs of abuse.*

Chapter 4

The Neuroscience of Cravings and Dependency

*"All these, and many others, have one symptom in common;
they cannot start drinking without developing the phenomenon of
craving.... They took a drink a day or so prior to the date, and
then the phenomenon of craving at once became paramount to all
other interests so that the important appointment was not met."*
~Excerpts from "The Doctor's Opinion," by Dr. Carl Jung,
basic text of the *Big Book of Alcoholics Anonymous*, 1939

Sheila M.: Loves to Party

Sheila M. is a fiftyish women married to the same man for twenty-plus
years with four children. Today Sheila lives a charmed life in the suburbs
of the Midwest. She was my classmate in college and, during her college
years, liked to party. I ran into her at a reunion function not long ago.
When in college she drank heavily, liked marijuana, hashish, and cocaine,
and did occasional LSD. She smoked tobacco and clove cigarettes. Pound
for pound, she "out-partied" most of the football players I knew. She
just liked to feel good; to "catch a buzz" and have a good time. When
she got pregnant with her first child in her late twenties, she stopped
everything. Sheila just stopped cold turkey. She said she had no significant
withdrawals or cravings. For the last twenty-five-plus years, she has drunk
socially, a cocktail or a glass of wine here and there. She never became an
"addict," according to the official DSM-IV definition. She is what all true
addicts and alcoholics yearn for: to be a recreational user of mood-altering

substances. She is in stark contrast to Clark A., a true addict whose story is presented at the end of the chapter.

Transition from Casual Use to Addiction

Scientists have agreed that drugs of abuse stimulate the common reward pathways in the brain. As with Sheila's case, not everyone who takes a mood-altering substance becomes an addict. *When the reward pathways are chronically stimulated by drugs of abuse, addiction often occurs, especially in those who are genetically or otherwise neurochemically vulnerable.* Activation of brain reward systems is generally a natural component of normal behavior. Indeed, brain reward systems serve to direct the organism's behavior toward goals that are normally beneficial and promote survival of the individual (e.g., food and water intake) or the species (e.g., reproductive behavior). Drugs of abuse not only stimulate areas of the brain that have evolved to encourage adaptive behaviors; they stimulate these areas more effectively than the survival behaviors themselves!

However, simple activation of brain reward systems does not constitute addiction. The key question in the study of addiction is why some individuals make the transition from casual or recreational drug use to compulsive use (addiction) whereas others do not. The following discussion summarizes our current knowledge of the changes that occur in nerve cells and their connections, in specific areas of our brains, during the pathological growth of the disease of addiction.

Neurobiology of Substance Dependence

Neurobiological accounts of drug addiction must account for behaviors and symptoms of the drug addict. The *Diagnostic and Statistical Manual of Mental Disorders* (DSM-IV) refers to drug addiction as *"substance dependence,"* the essential characteristic of which is a compulsive pattern of drug-seeking and drug-taking behavior that continues despite adverse consequences.

As many addicts will contend, one of the main reasons they continue with their addiction is the avoidance of withdrawal. According to the DSM IV, the symptom of *withdrawal* is prime characteristic of dependence. Withdrawal symptoms vary with the substance, but usually involve onerous negative somatic and affective symptoms (dysphoria) after discontinued use.

Substance dependence is also characterized by *"tolerance."* Tolerance refers to drug-induced adaptations that lead to diminishing effects of a constant drug dose. It is well-known, in the circles of addicts and alcoholics, the need for increasing doses of the drug of choice to produce the same effect as their disease progresses.

Drug dependence is also characterized by *"craving."* Cravings are the reverse of tolerance and refer to drug-induced adaptations that enhance drug responsiveness with repeated drug exposure and create a feeling of "wanting" in the absence of the drug. Craving has been explained in neurobiological terms as *"neural sensitization,"* which is expressed primarily during cue exposure or return to "experimental" drug usage after a period of abstinence (Chao and Nestler, 2004). *The process of neural sensitization is likely responsible for the phenomenon of craving referred to in the passage of Alcoholics Anonymous cited at the beginning of this chapter.*

There are three predominant theories in the literature that explain the compulsive behaviors of addiction: They are the (1) hedonic, (2) learning-based, and (3) incentive-sensitization theories (Robinson, 1993; Chao, 2004).

The hedonic theory characterizes the transition from casual drug use to addiction in terms of affective states, either positive or negative, as experienced by the individual. The basic tenet of this theory draws from the traditional view of addiction, in which initial drug-taking results in a positive affective state (e.g., euphoria or pleasure), but upon cessation of the drug a withdrawal reaction occurs, leading to a negative affective state (e.g. anhedonia or dysphoria). The addict, therefore, feels the need to alleviate this negative affective state by continued drug use, thus explaining the compulsive element of addiction. *According to this theory, as drug taking continues, the hedonic set point is raised (tolerance), and the same amount of drug results in weaker positive hedonic effects and stronger negative after-effects when the drug is withdrawn. The transition from the initial positive hedonic state to an increasing negative hedonic state draws the individual into a spiral of homeostatic deregulation of brain reward pathways, resulting in the development of addiction and vulnerability to relapse.* This state of chronic homeostatic deregulation is termed *"allostasis,"* defined as a state of progressive deviation of motivational regulatory systems by chronic drug use from their normal function, with the establishment of a new hedonic (pleasure/pain) set point.

Addictive drugs initially produce positive reinforcing effects from actions at the ventral tegmental area, the nucleus accumbens, and the amygdala. Activation of the mesocorticolimbic dopamine pathway is the primary route of positive reinforcement in addiction for psychostimulant drugs, but the opioid peptides (endorphins), serotonin, and gamma-aminobutyric acid (GABA) have key roles for other non-psychostimulant drugs. These so-called *"reward neurotransmitters"* induce hedonic effects of euphoria and a feeling of well-being.

Withdrawal from a drug of abuse induces symptoms of negative affect such as dysphoria, depression, irritability, and anxiety. Deregulation of brain reward systems involves some of the same neurochemical pathways implicated in the drug's acute reinforcing effects, but in this case, they represent an opponent or opposite process (Ingjaldsson, 2003; Altman, 1996). During acute abstinence, increases in brain reward thresholds (a higher set point for drug reward) are a consequence of reduced reward neurotransmitters. This in turn may contribute to the negative emotional state of withdrawal and vulnerability to relapse (Sinha, 2001). Neurochemical changes during opioid withdrawal include decreases in dopaminergic and serotonergic transmission and increased sensitivity of opioid receptor transduction mechanisms. Escalating doses of opioids, like those seen in the human pattern of morphine or heroin use, are associated with profound alterations in the function of mu-opioid receptors (O'Brien, 1998). A decrease in baseline reward mechanisms leads to an increase in drug intake to compensate for the shift in reward baseline (Wilson, 2004).

Stress response systems of the body also engage to contribute to the negative emotional state experienced with abstinence; these can exacerbate drug craving and seeking. Chronic drug use adversely affects the hypothalamic-pituitary-adrenal axis, disrupting regulation of hypothalamic corticotropin-releasing factor (CRF). Particularly important is activation of CRF in the extra-hypothalamic brain stress system, amygdala, and related structures. CRF controls hormonal, sympathetic, and behavioral responses to stress. During acute withdrawal of the drug, production of adrenocorticotropic hormone, cortisol, amygdala CRF, norepinephrine, and other neurotransmitters induce brain arousal, stress-like responses, and a dysphoric, aversive state. The activation and recruitment of brain and hormonal stress responses contribute to a deviation in brain reward set point (Wilson, 2004). *The stress response also is a source of negative reinforcement that leads to compulsive drug-seeking behavior.* (More about stress in Chapter 5.)

Learning-based theories of addiction propose that repeated drug exposure is associated with particularly strong memories, mediated by drug-induced changes in brain reward regions. Accordingly, drug taking is a learned response to conditioned stimuli, such as drug-associated cues (Littleton, 2002). The theory of "incentive sensitization" proposes a similar learning phenomenon, although draws a distinction between drug "liking" and drug "wanting." This theory proposes that the excessive "wanting" of the drug and the excessive incentive salience attached to drug-associated stimuli drives compulsive drug seeking, drug taking, and relapse (Tiffany, 1999). "Liking" refers to the feeling of the non-addict.

In learning-based theories, craving and relapse are predominantly explained as a process of associative learning, whereby environmental and emotional stimuli repeatedly paired with drug consumption acquire an incentive-motivational value, evoking expectation of drug availability and memories of past drug euphoria (Everitt, 2001). Conditioned responses to such stimuli can activate brain reward mechanisms that instigate craving. Functional brain imaging in humans (Daglish, 2003; Miller, 2001; Goldstein, 2002), as well as animal experiments (Everitt, 2001; See, 2002), have implicated interconnections between areas of the frontal cortex and the limbic system responsible for cravings. Major components of this neural circuitry include the orbitofrontal cortex, anterior cingulate, perilimbic cortex, basolateral amygdala, hippocampus, and nucleus accumbens.

Neuronal Changes with Chronic Drug Use

Chronic drug use induces changes in the structure and function of the central nervous system's neurons that last for years, if not a lifetime, after exposure to the drug. These adaptations account for both the tolerance and cravings characteristic of addiction. (Robinson and Berridge, 2003)

We can thank our friends in the animal kingdom that granted us the privilege to study their brains for this research. In multiple studies using rats and mice, researchers have shown that animals will self-administer the same substances that humans abuse—including cocaine, heroin, amphetamine and many other common habit-forming drugs. In these experiments, animals are given three options: (1) if they press lever A, they get an infusion of a drug through an IV; (2) if they press level B, they get an infusion of normal saline; and, (3), if they press lever C, they get a food pellet. Within a few days, a percentage of the animals will become addicted to the drug; they readily self-administer. Researchers have further observed that the animals display addictive behaviors. Addicted animals will self-administer drugs at the expense of normal activities, such as eating and sleeping; some die of exhaustion or malnutrition. Addicted animals have been observed to labor around the clock to obtain more, pressing a lever hundreds of times for a single dose. The animals also learn to associate particular details of their surroundings with acquisition of the drug (Guitart, 1992; Deroche, 2004). They prefer to be in areas in the cage where lever pressing had given them the drug, days after the drug has been taken away. This behavior is reminiscent of human addicts who experience cravings at the site of drug paraphernalia or liquor stores.

Months after the drug is removed from their environment, addicted rats will immediately return to its exhaustive bar-pressing behavior when given just a taste of the drug or placed in a cage it associates with a drug effect. When addicted rats are exposed to psychological stresses, such as foot shock, they engage in lever-pressing behavior for the drug (Sinha, 2001). Identical stimuli that are exposure to low doses of drug, drug-associated cues, and/or stress are known to trigger craving and relapse in human addicts. Through studying the behaviors and brains of these brave addicted animals, researchers have identified the areas of the brain involved in and the neural changes responsible for addiction.

CREB, Dynorphin and Delta FosB

We know from human experience that addiction is characterized by tolerance and dependence. So what have we learned from our animal studies about the changes that occur at the neuron level in addiction? Researchers have found that the state or condition of tolerance can be explained by the action of a small molecule known as CREB (cAMP response element-binding protein) (Lonze, 2002). CREB is a transcription factor, a protein that regulates the expression, or activity, of genes and thereby the overall behavior of nerve cells. Drugs of abuse stimulate dopamine release in the nucleus accumbens, which triggers production of a small signaling molecule, cyclic AMP (cAMP), which in turn activates CREB. CREB protein binds to specific genes, stimulating the production of proteins leading the changes in cellular function. Some of the proteins generated via CREB stimulation dampen the reward circuitry, perhaps in a protective fashion. Dynorphin is one of these proteins.

Dynorphin is a small protein with opiate-like effects synthesized by a subset of neurons in the nucleus accumbens (Newton, 2002; Shippenberg, 1997). These neurons send connections to and, through the action of dynorphin, inhibit neurons in the VTA. Production of dynorphin by CREB thereby dampens the brain's reward circuitry, creating the state of tolerance—that is, more drug is needed for the same effect. Dynorphin is also hypothesized to be responsible for dependence and withdrawal, as its inhibition of the reward pathway leaves the individual, in the drug's absence, in a state of dysphoria or depression, unable to take pleasure in previously enjoyable activities.

The CREB transcription factor is switched off after a few days, so this factor cannot alone be accountable for the risk of relapse which is known to be seen in addicts and alcoholics and can last years or decades after abstinence. Other brain alterations must be occurring. Researchers have termed these neural alterations as *"sensitization,"* a phenomenon whereby the effects of a drug are augmented, even after prolonged abstinence. Days after discontinuing drug usage, CREB activity declines, CREB-induced tolerance wanes, and sensitization engages. Sensitization is accountable for the intense craving experienced by a drug user at the mere taste or memory of the drug. Scientists have found another transcription factor, delta FosB, which turns on for months after cessation of drug use and is accountable for changes in the morphology of neurons (Chao and Nestler, 2004).

Researchers have shown in mice and rats that, in response to chronic drug abuse, delta FosB concentrations rise gradually and progressively in the nucleus accumbens and other brain regions. The protein is relatively large and stable and remains active in these nerve cells for weeks to months after drug administration, enabling it to maintain changes in gene expression for months after cessation of the drug. *Drug-addicted mice that produce excessive amounts of delta FosB in the nucleus accumbens become hypersensitive to drugs. These mice were highly prone to relapse after the drugs were withdrawn and later made available.*

Delta FosB is hypothesized to be, at least in part, responsible for the morphological changes seen in the nerve cells of the nucleus accumbens of drug-addicted rats. These nerve cells are known as medium spiny neurons and show morphological changes long after delta FosB levels have returned to normal. In addicted animals medium spiny neurons in the nucleus accumbens show additional branches (dendrites) and synaptic connections; therefore, every time they are stimulated there is a significant increase in dopamine release compared with normal neurons. The signal between nerve cells is amplified in proportion to the number of additional connections, as well as the strength of these connections. In rodents, researchers have found that these additional branches and connections continue for months after the cessation of drug taking. Researchers hypothesize that it is the heightened signaling that causes the addict's brain to overreact to drug-related cues. The dendritic changes are likely the central nervous system's way of adapting to the overstimulation produced by drugs of abuse.

Neural Sensitization

Along with transcription factor delta FosB, studies have implicated other proteins, called *"neurotrophic factors,"* which can control neuronal morphology and function, in drug addiction. Several recent studies have implicated that neurotrophic factors mediate plasticity in the adult nervous system via their ability to regulate synaptic transmission as well as maintain growth, survival, and differentiation of neurons (Thoenen, 1995). Dopaminergic neurons of the VTA produce brain-derived neurotrophic factor (BDNF) and neurotrophin 3 (NT3) as well as several receptor proteins. Similarly, medium spiny neurons of the NA produce TrkB and TrkC receptor proteins as well as low levels of BDNF (Pierce, 2001). Researchers agree that the details of the mechanics of dendritic growth and synaptic potentiation remain mysterious and an area of active investigation.

Associative Learning and the Extended Limbic System

Although the VTA-NA circuit is a key detector of rewarding stimuli, other areas of the brain, involved in associative learning, have been found to be recruited in the addicted brain. The *amygdala* is particularly important for conditioned aspects of drug exposure—for example, establishing associations between environmental cues and both the rewarding actions of acute drug exposure and the aversive symptoms during drug withdrawal. The *hippocampus*, the hub of the memory circuit, is crucial for memory formation of the context of drug exposure and withdrawal. The *hypothalamus* is important in mediating many effects of drugs on the body's physiological state, particularly the stress responses.

Probably most important are the roles of certain areas of the frontal lobe, such as the medial prefrontal cortex, anterior cingulate cortex, and orbitofrontal cortex. *These regions provide executive control over drug use, which is severely impaired in many addicts.* Of course, these brain regions, and many more, do not function separately, but are parts of a complex and highly integrated circuit that is profoundly altered by drug exposure.

The Phenomenon of Craving

Several researchers have studied the phenomenon of craving and its role in relapse, the return to drug use after a period of abstinence. *Critical for craving and relapse is the process of associative learning, whereby environmental stimuli repeatedly paired with drug consumption acquire incentive/motivational value, evoking memories of past drug euphoria* (Littleton, 2000; See, 2002; Everitt, 2001). Classic conditioned responses to internal or external stimuli can activate brain reward mechanisms and have been implicated by several authors as being integral to the phenomenon of craving (Kenny, 2003; Drummond, 2001; Tiffany, 2000).

In humans, the phenomenon of craving is difficult to measure, although functional brain imaging studies have identified brain regions activated in response to drug cues. In animals, however, behavioral reactivity to drug cues can be studied directly. Functional brain imaging in humans (Daglish, 2003; Miller, 2001; Goldstein, 2002) and lesion and site-specific pharmacological manipulations in animals (Cardinal, 2002) have implicated an interconnected set of cortical and limbic brain regions in associative learning underlying craving and relapse. Major components of this circuitry include the orbitofrontal cortex (OFC), anterior cingulate cortex (ACC), prefrontal cortex (PFC), amygdala, hippocampus, nucleus accumbens, and more recently, dorsal striatum.

The OFC and PFC have been found to modulate cocaine-seeking in rodents and subregions have been identified—with the lateral orbitofrontal cortex involved in conditioned stimuli response and the medial orbitofrontal cortex involved in the "priming response" (Fuchs, 2004; Franklin, 2002; Schoenbaum, 2004; Volkow, 2000) Considering the "executive function" of the PFC that includes risk-benefit analysis and suppression of limbic impulses, the shift in activation of the PFC could contribute to impaired impulse control, and lack of judgment and risk assessment, which are defining features of addictive behavior (Bechara, 1994). Animal studies have revealed that the learned responses to drug cues and the induction of cue-induced cravings is modulated by glutaminergic connections from the PFC, OFC, and ACC to the VTA and NA.

In addicted animals, the sensitivity of the reward pathway to glutamate stimulation from the aforementioned frontal lobe areas is increased, resulting in both the release of dopamine from the VTA and responsiveness to dopamine in the NA, thereby promoting CREB and delta FosB activity and their neuroadaptive effects. This altered glutamate-modulated sensitivity strengthens neural pathways and reinforces the link memories of drug-taking experiences and reward, thereby initiating drug-seeking behavior. The exact mechanism by which drugs alter sensitivity to glutamate in neurons of the reward pathway is not yet known with certainty. It is a working hypothesis that glutamate affects neurons in the hippocampus, the center of memory in the limbic system. The phenomenon called *"long-term potentiation"* has been described for the formation of memories, whereby short-term stimuli or events are recorded in a nerve cell's synapse for hours to decades. With long-term potentiation, glutamate-binding receptor proteins are transported from intracellular stores to the cell membrane, where they can be readily available to glutamate released into the synapse. Through long-term potentiation, the glutamate receptors are strengthened; their response is amplified with each stimulus. These neuroplastic changes are brought about by repeated exposure to drugs and are relatively permanent.

Mechanisms of Effect of Individual Drugs of Abuse

Alcohol

Alcohol is classified as a depressant. Alcohol deserves separate mention, however, because of its effect on multiple neurotransmitters and cell membrane integrity in general (Bakalkin, 2008). The chemistry of ethanol is relevant to an understanding of the neurobiology of alcohol addiction. Ethyl alcohol (ethanol) is a small organic molecule consisting of a two-carbon backbone surrounded by hydrogen atoms, with a hydroxyl group attached to one of these carbons. The hydroxyl group provides ethanol with its water-soluble properties, while the hydrocarbon backbone gives ethanol some of its lipid-soluble properties. This composition of ethanol gives it the capacity to interact with and dissolve into both water and lipid. This amphiphilic property of ethanol has been a major impetus for the hypotheses that try to define ethanol's mechanism of action through the perturbation of cell membranes. This perturbation of the membrane of the neuron is theorized to result in the functional changes seen during alcoholic intoxication.

This *"membrane hypothesis"* of ethanol's actions may also explain the high-dose anesthetic effects of ethanol. However, the lower-dose effects—which include reinforcement, anxiolytic effects, motor incoordination, and cognitive effects, as well as the development of tolerance and dependence—are not as easily related to ethanol-induced perturbation of cell membranes. The current conceptualization is that the lower-dose effects of ethanol are mediated through the interaction of ethanol with a specific subset of neuronal elements (receptors, enzymes, etc.) that are particularly sensitive to ethanol (Tabakoff and Hoffman, 1992). The most recent findings support the hypothesis that alcohol produces its effects by intercollating itself into membranes, resulting in increased fluidity of the membrane with short-term exposure to ethanol. It is also theorized that long-term use of ethanol results in membrane stiffness (Raitses, 2010). It has long been known that membrane fluidity is critical to the normal functioning of receptors, ion channels, and other membrane processes

The acute effects of alcohol on the brain result mainly from its effects on the postsynaptic receptor sites for various neurotransmitters (Paul, 2006). The depressant effects of alcohol arise from its action on GABA receptors, the principal postsynaptic receptors for the inhibitory neurotransmitter GABA. When stimulated by GABA, these receptors respond by opening an ion channel that allows chloride ions to enter the neuron, which hyperpolarizes the membrane and reduces the chance for an action potential to occur. The receptors are sensitive to alcohol, enhancing the inhibiting effects of GABA.

However, the effects of the chronic use of alcohol are quite different, and result in a decreased sensitivity of GABA receptors to both alcohol and GABA itself. Alcohol appears to actually change genetic expression of the neuron and thus change the structure of the receptor proteins generated by the cell. This manifests itself as increased tolerance to the effects of alcohol, since more of the drug is required to achieve the same depressant and intoxicating effect. Because of the damage to the function of the GABA inhibitory system, the central nervous system (CNS) tends toward hyperexcitability, resulting in anxiety, tremors, disorientation, and hallucinations associated with alcohol withdrawal. Chronic exposure to alcohol may also increase the sensitivity of glutamate receptors, and since glutamate is an excitatory neurotransmitter, this would contribute further to CNS hyperexcitability.

Alcohol also seems to affect the binding properties of receptors for opioid peptides, as well as the synthesis of these peptides. Specifically, alcohol may stimulate the release of beta-endorphins, neurotransmitters held responsible for euphoria and anesthesia, accounting for some of the intoxicating effects of alcohol (Graham, 1998). The experimental observation that the administration of opioid blockers reduces craving for alcohol has led to FDA approval of naltrexone, a drug that interferes with the function of opioid receptors, as a treatment for alcoholism.

Through alterations in GABA and opiate receptor activity, alcohol affects the limbic dopamine reward system (Hoffman, 1996). GABA and the opioid peptide neurotransmitters are active in the reward system and play a role in regulating dopamine (reward) secretion. Alcohol, whether directly or indirectly through its effects on the receptors of neurotransmitters affecting the dopaminergic system, causes an increase in the amount of dopamine released in the limbic system. The neurotransmitter, serotonin, present in the hypothalamus, also seems to affect the system by regulating the activity of dopamine (Oscar-Berman, 2003). Therefore, alcohol, unlike other receptor-specific drugs, affects multiple neurotransmitter systems.

Depressants

Depressants reduce the activity of a specific part of the brain. Depressants often are referred to as "downers" due to their dampening or "downing" effects. Depressants are widely used throughout the world as prescription medicines and as illicit substances. When these are used, effects may include anxiolysis, analgesia, sedation, somnolence, cognitive/memory impairment, dissociation, muscle relaxation, lowered blood pressure/heart rate, respiratory depression, anesthesia, and anticonvulsant effects. Some are also capable of inducing feelings of euphoria. Anesthetics, sedatives, tranquillizers and alcohol are examples of depressants.

Depressants exert their effects through a number of different pharmacological mechanisms, the most prominent of which include facilitation of GABA and/or opioid activity, and inhibition of stimulatory, adrenergic or acetylcholine, activity. Depressants such as barbiturates and benzodiazepines, work by increasing the affinity of the GABA receptor for its ligand, GABA. The GABA effects on neural transmission are complex and beyond the scope of this text. Narcotics such as morphine and heroin, work by mimicking endorphins (chemicals produced naturally by the body and have effects similar to dopamine) or disabling the neurons that normally inhibit the release of dopamine in the reward system. These substances typically facilitate relaxation and pain relief.

Opiates

Opiates are a highly addictive set of drugs that include opium, morphine, and heroin. All of these drugs come from the same plant, the opium poppy. In Asia, opium is usually smoked as a powder or pulp that is derived easily from the poppy seeds. Morphine is a much more potent synthesis of the poppy seed which was developed as a pain medication by the military so that people who had severe injuries might be comforted. One of the most popular opiates is heroin, a drug used around the world for its euphoric and calming effects. Heroin is highly addictive and has a very painful physical withdrawal syndrome, making it hard to quit. Studying the opiates' effect on the brain led to important discoveries in the natural process of pain control and our understanding of our sense of well-being.

Opiates are neurotransmitter-like substances that fit very well into certain endorphin receptor sites. These receptor sites were discovered through the action of opiates, even before discovery of the natural substance meant for these receptors. Finally, endorphins, such as enkephalin, were identified as a primary natural substance that helps us cope with pain and critical stress. Actually, the endorphins our bodies produce are very much like opiates. They can create euphoric-like states and are now being identified as the "natural opiates." Endorphins can be produced within our body by those behaviors closely related to the fight-or-flight syndrome. At the first sign of danger, our body will start producing endorphins.

The brain circuits involved in opiate reinforcement appear to be very similar to that mediating cocaine self-administration (Johnson, 1992). Limbic structures are clearly implicated in opiate reinforcement, but a central role for dopamine is less obvious. Significant changes in the utilization of some chemicals (neurotransmitters) involved in transmission between brain cells have been shown in the nucleus accumbens, amygdala, and frontal and cingulate cortices of animals intravenously self-administering morphine. Similarly, nucleus-accumbens dopamine does not appear to be elevated as significantly in animals self-administering heroin as it is in animals self-administering cocaine. However, evidence does indicate an important role for limbic structures and chemicals used to communicate between cells of the limbic system in opiate reinforcement.

Stimulants

Stimulants, such as amphetamines, nicotine, and cocaine, increase dopamine signaling in the reward system either by directly stimulating its release, or by blocking its absorption. These substances (sometimes called "uppers") typically cause heightened alertness and energy. They cause a pleasant feeling in the body and euphoria, known as a high. Once this high wears off, the user may feel depressed. This makes them want another dose of the drug, and can worsen the addiction.

Amphetamines, cocaine, and nicotine are the three common drugs that actually increase the neurotransmitter, dopamine, in the brain. These drugs are considered stimulants. The problem with this otherwise advantageous effect is that when dopamine is released beyond natural homeostatic protection of the endocrine system, the body is not allowed to sleep or rest. The brain needs to go through its normal cycle of conscious states. If it becomes forced by continuous stimulants to bypass the states achieved during rest and sleep, the brain will force the issue. When this happens, the individual will begin to have waking dreams, a state almost identical to psychosis. Unconscious and extremely violent behavior is often exhibited.

Amphetamines and cocaine act on the individual, like tobacco, by increasing our neural activity, endurance, and stamina. The effects of cocaine and nicotine last a very short time and become very addictive through their stimulation of the limbic dopamine reward system. The brain is well motivated to continue this stimulation, but the uninterrupted use of these drugs tends to lead to serious social and psychological problems, which include psychosis and violent behaviors.

Amphetamines were used in this country as diet pills for many years before being banned by the FDA. Cocaine is native to the mountains of South America, where it is chewed by the indigenous people who carry their agricultural products to market on foot over steep terrain. The cocaine plant is a perfect source of high non-caloric energy for extended endurance and stamina. If the natural plant is chewed and the stomach is allowed to regulate absorption, the euphoric effects of the processed version used by addicts are not experienced.

Marijuana

Marijuana is often mistakenly grouped with hallucinogenics. It is best described as a sedative hypnotic. The active ingredient of cannabis is Δ^9-tetrahydrocannabinol (Delta^9-THC) and it is thought to exert its effect by binding to cannabinoid (CB1) receptors on pre-synaptic nerve terminals in the brain. Delta^9-THC binding to CB1 receptors activates "G-proteins" which activate/inhibit a number of signal transduction pathways in the limbic reward centers. The cumulative effect of these pathways is the euphoric feelings associated with cannabis use.

Other reported effects include relaxation, altered space-time perception, alteration of visual, auditory, and olfactory senses, disorientation, fatigue, and appetite stimulation (colloquially known as "the munchies"). The mechanism for appetite stimulation in subjects is believed to result from activity in the hypothalamus. Hunger centers in the hypothalamus increase the desirability of food when levels of a hunger hormone, ghrelin, increase as food enters the stomach. Cannabinoid activity is reduced through the satiety signals induced by leptin release. THC has anti-emetic effects, promoting its medicinal use in patients receiving chemotherapy. THC has mild-to-moderate analgesic effects and can be used to treat mild-to-moderate pain. The mechanism for analgesic effects caused directly by THC or other cannabinoid agonists is not fully understood.

Hallucinogenics

Hallucinogenics are different in the sense that they seem to produce effects similar to psychotic episodes (Sullivan, 2002). They work on areas of the brain related more specifically to perception and symbolic reasoning. These drugs include hundreds of naturally occurring substances and include plants of many species. Cacti, mushrooms, and wild herbs are the most commonly known.

LSD binds to and activates a specific receptor for the neurotransmitter serotonin. Normally, serotonin binds to and activates its receptors, and then is taken back up into the neuron that released it. In contrast, LSD binds very tightly to the serotonin receptor, causing a greater than normal activation of the receptor. Because serotonin has a role in many of the brain's functions, activation of its receptors by LSD produces widespread effects, including rapid emotional swings, altered perceptions, and if taken in a large enough dose, delusions and visual hallucinations.

PCP (phencyclidine), which is not a true hallucinogen, can affect many neurotransmitter systems (Gorelick, 2010). It interferes with the functioning of the neurotransmitter glutamate, which is found in neurons throughout the brain. Like many other drugs, it causes dopamine to be released from neurons into the synapse. At low-to-moderate doses, PCP causes altered perception of body image, but rarely produces visual hallucinations. PCP can also cause effects that mimic the primary symptoms of schizophrenia, such as delusions and mental turmoil. People who use PCP for long periods of time have memory loss and speech difficulties. PCP is a three-ringed molecule that is structurally similar to ketamine. However, PCP differs from ketamine in that it is longer acting, is more likely to cause seizures, and tends to cause more emergent confusion and delirium.

PCP is a noncompetitive antagonist at the glutamate NMDA receptor and binds to sites located in the cortex and limbic structures of the brain. This mechanism is believed to be responsible for most of the dissociative effects of PCP. PCP has been shown to affect biogenic amine (e.g., dopamine, norepinephrine, and serotonin) release and reuptake in a dose-dependent manner. These actions may account for the sympathomimetic effects after PCP ingestion. In addition, PCP may indirectly modulate cholinergic and GABAergic outflow in the CNS.

Designer drugs

Designer drugs (sometimes referred to as "club drugs") are a particular class of synthetic drugs most often associated with underground youth dance parties called 'raves' (Henderson, 1988). These drugs have been created by changing the molecular structure of other existing drugs, to create something new with similar pharmacological effects—hence, the name "designer drug." They are plentiful, cheap and dangerous. For example, the pharmaceutical drug fentanyl (which was originally created as an anesthetic) has been modified to be 80 to 1,000 times more potent than heroin. Some designer drugs, like GHB, are depressants, so they are used when an individual is "coming down" from a stimulant like Ecstasy. Two of the most popular designer drugs are MDMA (or 'Ecstasy') and ketamine (or 'Special K')

The mechanism of action of MDMA is incompletely understood, but it is believed to inhibit the reuptake of serotonin (5-HT), to facilitate serotonin release, and to a lesser extent cause dopamine and noradrenaline. The serotonin boost can produce a sense of emotional closeness, elation, and sensory delight. MDMA acute adverse effects may include increased heart rate and blood pressure, tremor, sweating, bruxism, and life-threatening hyperthermia that may be further complicated by rhabdomyolysis (muscle breakdown), disseminated intravascular coagulation, and acute renal failure.

Ketamine molecular structure and mechanism of action are similar to those of PCP. It acts as a noncompetitive antagonist on the NMDA receptor. The drug's secondary interactions with muscarinic, nicotinic, and cholinergic receptors inhibit the neuronal uptake of norepinephrine, dopamine, and serotonin. At high doses, ketamine binds to mu and sigma opioid receptors, which are thought to be responsible for the loss of consciousness under controlled anesthesia. It also lowers the heart rate, so it can lead to oxygen starvation to the brain and muscles. An overdose can also cause the heart to stop. Like most anesthetics, eating or drinking before taking ketamine may cause vomiting. Temporary paralysis has been reported in some users but is rare.

Brain Imaging Studies of Addiction

The results from recent neuroimaging studies and the learning-based theory of addiction have implicated additional brain areas other than the limbic reward centers involved in addiction. This makes sense. *Neuroanatomists have long recognized the rich communication between the limbic centers and the perilimbic cortices.* The perilimbic cortices are notably in the frontal lobe, which is inclusive of the cingulate gyrus, orbitofrontal and prefrontal cortex; and temporal lobe, inclusive of the insular cortex and parahippocampal gyrus.

Numerous neuroimaging studies have implicated the frontal cortex as being intimately involved in the addictive process. This implies that dopamine involvement in drug addiction involves dopaminergic circuits from the limbic system to the frontal cortex. In support of this suggestion are the findings of several recent structural/volumetric MRI studies documenting morphological changes in the frontal lobe in chronic drug addiction. Frontal lobe volume losses have been identified in alcoholic subjects (Jerrigan, 1991; Pfefferbaum, 1997), cocaine-dependent subjects (Liu, 1998; Franklin, 2002), and polysubstance abuse subjects (Liu, 1998). These studies have implied a cumulative effect of substance abuse on frontal volumes.

Similar observations have been made in animals. For example, it has been recently shown that self-administration of cocaine, but not food, results in morphological changes in dendrites and dendritic spines in the prefrontal cortex and nucleus accumbens in rats (Robinson, 2001). In rats administered amphetamines, researchers observed suppression of the inhibition of the amygdala by the medial prefrontal cortex, possibly leading to a disinhibition of emotional responses, such as rage and fear (Rosenkranz, 2001). A similar process is very likely occurring in human drug addiction. *There is abundant evidence that the executive, supervisory functions of the frontal cortex are down regulated in human drug addiction, releasing emotions that are normally kept under close monitoring and suppressed.* Frontal lobe down-regulation means that previously unimpeded, well-conceived behaviors default to automatic sensory-driven paradigms with attribution of primary motivational salience to the drug of abuse at the expense of other available rewarding stimuli (or responsibilities).

In addition to the frontal cortex, several studies have also implicated the anterior insular cortex of the temporal lobe in drug addiction, particularly the phenomenon of craving. Research has shown that drug craving may be a particular instance of the anterior insula's broader role in interoception and subjective feeling states similar, for example, to thirst and hunger. An important role for the insula in craving is supported by evidence of insular activity changing with satiety and with the top–down cognitive modulation of cravings. The anterior insula has been implicated in a range of emotional processes, including representing visceral states (particularly those that give rise to emotional experiences), detecting discrepancies between one's expected and actual bodily arousal levels, in empathy, in processing decision-making related uncertainty, and in conscious awareness of one's bodily states (Craig, 2009; Hester, 2005; Singer, 2009; Paulus, 2006). Ma and colleagues (2010) recently reported increased resting-state connectivity between the left lateral orbitofrontal cortex and the left insula in heroin users relative to controls. Consistent with this, tracer studies in macaque monkeys have revealed strong afferent projections from the insula to the ventral striatum, which are thought to integrate consummatory behaviors with rewards and memory (Fudge,

2005). In addition to the insula, craving-related activations are often observed in the dorsolateral prefrontal, medial prefrontal, and orbitofrontal cortices, anterior and posterior cingulate cortex, ventral striatum, and amygdala.

Craving

Drug craving can be described as the subjective experience of an intense desire for a substance of abuse. Craving involves anticipation, euphoria, drive, appetite, shifted attention, and conditioned emotional responses but may or may not result in drug use intention or behavior. Craving is difficult to measure objectively. Researchers have used "cue reactivity" to study the phenomenon of craving. Cue reactivity is the response to a cue that has been classically conditioned with drug effects and is an observable event that modestly correlates with self-reports of craving (Tiffany, 2000). Cue reactivity has been demonstrated in alcohol dependent adults (Monti, 1987, 2000; Rohsenow, 1992) in the form of physiological changes, such as heart rate elevations or salivation to alcohol-related words, pictures, scents, tactile cues, or imaginary stimuli (McCusker, 1995; Monti, 1987; Stormark, 2000).

Brain functional magnetic resonance imaging (fMRI) studies have the power to reveal cognitive processes by measuring the metabolic activity of subcentimeter areas of the brain. In a study by Wrase (2007), sixteen detoxified male alcoholics and sixteen age-matched healthy volunteers participated in two fMRI paradigms. In the first paradigm, alcohol-associated and affectively neutral pictures were presented, whereas in the second paradigm, a monetary gain task was performed, in which brain activation during anticipation of monetary gain and loss was examined. For both paradigms, they assessed the association of alcohol craving with neural activation to incentive cues. Detoxified alcoholics showed reduced activation of the ventral striatum during anticipation of monetary gain relative to healthy controls, despite similar performance. However, alcoholics showed increased ventral striatal activation in response to alcohol-associated cues. Reduced activation in the ventral striatum during expectation of monetary reward, and increased activation during presentation of alcohol cues were correlated with alcohol craving in alcoholics, but not healthy controls.

In a recent study, comparing fMRI responses with visual alcohol cues in heavy drinkers compared with light drinkers, researchers found that when participants were confronted with visual cues related to alcohol, heavy drinkers showed amplified activity in specific emotional areas (insular cortex) and in parts of the brain's reward circuitry (ventral striatum) (Ihssen, 2010). This neuronal amplification was not present in light drinkers. Crucially, in the same imaging period, heavy drinkers showed reduced responses in the frontal cortex to pictures related to higher order life goals and in the cingulate cortex to appetitive food stimuli, suggesting that they have difficulty finding alternative, socially desirable goals other than alcohol. Using discriminant function analysis, they demonstrated that the combination of alcohol-related over activation and under activation to alternative goals allows heavy and light drinkers to be differentiated with a high degree of precision. *These results suggest that mesolimbic activation in alcoholics is biased toward processing rewarding alcoholic cues. This might explain why alcoholics find it particularly difficult to focus on natural rewarding activities, such as activities necessary for holding a job or maintaining a healthy family.*

There are several neuroimaging studies of craving for stimulants, which have produced remarkably consistent results. Researchers using glucose metabolites in PET imaging first showed that craving for cocaine correlated with increased metabolic activity in the amygdala and dorsolateral prefrontal cortex (Grant, 1996). Also using glucose metabolite PET imaging, Childress (1999) similarly showed that cocaine craving was associated with increased activity in the amygdala, but also in the anterior cingulate cortex. Previous studies have implicated the amygdala in associative learning (distinguishing good and bad), the anterior cingulate cortex with emotional processing and the dorsolateral prefrontal cortex with memory formation. Functional MRI studies have shown activation in similar areas in response to drug cues in abstinent addicts, including the anterior cingulate, prefrontal and orbitofrontal cortices (Wexler, 2001; Garavan, 2000).

Excellent experiments exploiting the power of fMRI have been used by Breiter (1997) to map the distinct regional effects of cocaine on the brain and relate these with subjective states. They found that the "rush" was associated with activation in areas including the basal forebrain, caudate, cingulate, and prefrontal cortices, whereas activation associated with craving occurred in the nucleus accumbens, right parahippocampal gyrus (near the insular cortex), and prefrontal cortex.

Several researchers have also identified the insula to be activated in drug craving (Craig 2009). For example, Naqvi and Bechara (2009) list sixteen studies reporting insula activation during drug urges in cigarette, cocaine, alcohol, and heroin users. More recently, marijuana craving has also been observed to produce insula activity (Filbey, 2009). In a direct test of the specificity of insular activity for cocaine craving, Garavan, et al. (2000) showed that insular activity of cocaine addicts, when viewing a video of cocaine use was also present when those users viewed a video containing erotic content and was also present when cocaine-naive controls viewed the erotic video. That said, the magnitude of responses to drug and non-drug stimuli in a common circuitry may be important.

There are only a handful of studies on opiate craving, but their results are similar to stimulants, supporting the hypothesis that there is a common pathway involved in addiction for drugs of abuse. Researchers reported that increased cerebral blood flow in the anterior cingulate cortex was seen in response to the salient drug cue, whereas craving itself was associated with activation in the left orbitofrontal cortex using PET imaging. These findings are similar to those using stimulants. Sell (2000) used similar paradigms to show "urge to use" or "craving" correlated strongly with increase cerebral blood flow in the inferior frontal and orbitofrontal cortices. Therefore, the orbitofrontal cortex appears to be associated with craving.

Perhaps related to the distinction between cue reactivity and craving, some studies have observed that brain responses to the initial period of exposure to drug stimuli (e.g., the first thirty seconds of a cocaine video) are more sensitive at discriminating users from controls (Kosten, 2006). Coupled with this is the evidence that limbic reactivity to drug stimuli can be induced by drug-related stimuli that are not consciously perceived (Childress, 2008) and theories of drug dependence that suggest that habitual or automatic behavioral repertoires might suffice to maintain dependence (Tiffany 1990; Everitt, 2005). In this regard, craving-related activations are consistently observed in the dorsolateral prefrontal, medial prefrontal, and orbitofrontal cortex, anterior and posterior cingulate cortex, ventral striatum, insula, and amygdala.

Brain Regions Activated by Craving

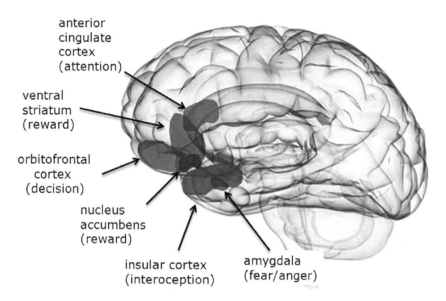

anterior
cingulate
cortex
(attention)

ventral
striatum
(reward)

orbitofrontal
cortex
(decision)

nucleus
accumbens
(reward)

insular cortex
(interoception)

amygdala
(fear/anger)

Heinz, et al. (2009) reported that a larger ventral striatal fMRI response to alcohol-related stimuli predicted higher relapse rates in alcoholics, whereas a larger response to non-drug, affectively-positive stimuli predicted a lower relapse rate. Curiously, in a task showing drug-related stimuli, Grusser et al. (2004) found that activity in response to alcohol-related stimuli in the putamen, anterior cingulate, and medial prefrontal cortex, but not the insula, predicted relapse. Here, subjective craving was also a poor predictor, which may suggest that an insula-mediated craving response is not the most sensitive in predicting relapse.

Both hunger and thirst have been shown to activate the insula (Del Parigi, 2002; Egan, 2003; Tataranni, 1999). Using the combination of a monotonous dietary manipulation and a cue-induction technique, robust caudate, hippocampal, and insular activity was observed as subjects imagined their favorite foods (Pelchat, 2004). Using a five-hour fasting manipulation, pictures of foods activated orbitofrontal cortex and bilateral insula with the insula activity correlating with subjective ratings of appetite (Porubska, 2006). In support of the insula's role in craving, Volkow et al. (2010) reported that cognitive inhibition of a video-induced craving response in cocaine abusers resulted in suppression of metabolism in the right posterior insula. In addition, Wang et al. (2009) reported that men, but not women, who inhibited their desire for food showed a corresponding reduction in metabolic activity in the insula. (By the way, those with insular lesions do not lose weight.)

Further insight into the neurobiology of drug craving has been gained by looking at variations in magnitude of cravings. This has been done experimentally by, for example, manipulating levels of cue or drug exposure or by exploiting variation in craving over time. Risinger et al. (2005) employed a self-administration procedure wherein cocaine addicts were able to self-administer up to six intravenous injections of cocaine within a one-hour fMRI session. The addicts were also able to provide frequent subjective reports of their feelings using Likert feeling scales throughout the imaging session. Utilizing the subjective ratings of the drug addict enables researchers to track the brain regions that correspond to the powerful experiences induced by the drug self-administrations. It was found that the time course of subjective "high" ratings correlated positively with right insular activity. At the same time, the reported subjective high across the study was inversely correlated with the time-course of subjective craving. The significant positive correlation between the insula and high might also reflect a negative relationship between insula activity and subjective craving. The authors conclude that the positive correlation between the insula and high suggests that the feelings associated with the drug high overwhelm any relationship between insula activity and craving.

Acute Intoxication

Several brain neuroimaging studies have assessed the effects of acute drug administration and intoxication on functional brain activity, such as glucose metabolism, cerebral blood flow, and oxygen utilization. These studies have revealed some interesting and some inconsistent findings. This is likely due to the degree of intoxication, and the development of concurrent cravings, relative tolerance of individuals studied, as well as minor differences in study protocols.

Several studies have shown lower glucose metabolism throughout the brain, including the frontal cortex, during cocaine, morphine, or alcohol intoxication (Volkow, 1990, London, 1990, deWitt, 1990). Alternatively, increased metabolism has been shown in the prefrontal cortex, anterior cingulate, orbitofrontal cortex, and striatum in cocaine abusers after sequential administration of intravenous methylphenidate, a cocaine analog (Volkow, 1999). The researchers observed that activation in the orbitofrontal cortex was only seen in the subjects in whom methylphenidate induced intense craving, and in the prefrontal cortex in the subjects in which it enhanced mood. Similarly, studies have shown that marijuana intoxication is associated with higher levels of glucose metabolism in the prefrontal cortex, orbitofrontal cortex, and striatum in marijuana abusers, but not in non-abusers (Volkow, 1996).

Studies measuring the effects of short-term drug administration on cerebral blood flow have consistently reported higher levels of prefrontal cerebral blood flow during intoxication with nicotine (Nakamura, 2000), marijuana (Mathew,1992), and alcohol (Volkow, 1988; Tihonen, 1994, Ingvar, 1998). Researchers observed that activation of the right prefrontal cortex during alcohol intoxication was associated with euphoria (Tihonen, 1994). Others demonstrated similar increases in prefrontal cortex blood flow during marijuana intoxication associated with the subjective sense of intoxication (Matthew, 1992). In contrast, studies of cerebral blood flow show that cocaine reduces blood flow throughout the brain, including the frontal cortex, an effect that could be attributed to cocaine's vasoconstricting effects (Wallace, 1996).

Functional MRI studies of oxygen utilization of the brain during various tasks show increased oxygen utilization within, or "activation" of the prefrontal cortex and anterior cingulate gyrus during cocaine intoxication, an effect that has been strongly correlated with drug reinforcement properties (Breiter, 1997). Researchers have shown that nicotine administration activates the frontal cortex and anterior cingulate gyrus, coinciding with the subjective experience of a "rush" and a "high" (Stein, 1998).

The discrepancies in activation patterns we see in these studies reflect the fact that different drugs have different vasoactive and drug-specific effects, and there are differences in the temporal course of biological phenomena measured (metabolism studies, thirty minutes to an hour; CBF studies, sixty seconds; oxygen utilization studies, three to five seconds). Since the metabolism and CBF (cerebral blood flow) studies are limited by showing processes that take hours to take effect, the functional MRI oxygen utilization methods best show drug-induced fast behavioral effects, such as a relatively rapid "rush" and "high."

Two studies have examined the effect on the brain of an acute dose of opiates. In one study, the effects of the short-acting opiate analog, fentanyl, was studied. In acutely intoxicated individuals, there was significantly increased activity in cingulate, orbitofrontal and medial prefrontal cortices, as well as the caudate nuclei (Firestone, 1996). These areas are involved in learning, reward, and addiction. In another study, using cerebral blood flow SPECT (single-photon emission computed tomography) imaging compared the effects of hydromorphone, an agonist at the mu receptor, which is responsible for the pleasurable effects of opiates, with those of butorphanol, an agonist at the kappa-opioid receptor, which mediates dysphoria. Hydromorphone, but not butorphanol, induced more euphoric effects and produced significant increases in activity in the anterior cingulate cortex, amygdala, and thalamus.

To summarize, the majority of the studies show activation in the prefrontal cortex and anterior cingulate gyrus during drug intoxication when using either the cerebral blood flow or functional MRI oxygen utilization methods. Prefrontal activation appears to be associated with the subjective perception of intoxication, the reinforcing effects of the drug, or enhanced mood.

The fact that, in the cases of marijuana or methylphenidate, the activation of the frontal regions was predominantly observed in the abusers but not in the non-abusing subjects suggests that prefrontal regions and the anterior cingulate are involved in the intoxication process and that their response to drugs is in part related to the reinforcing effects of previous drug experiences (Goldstein, 2002). Studies showing lower glucose metabolism throughout the brain, including the frontal, during cocaine, morphine, or alcohol intoxication are likely due to the overlapping of chronic changes or partial withdrawal effects and/or the effects of the vasoconstrictive effects of stimulant drugs (Volkow, 1990, London, 1990; de Witt, 1990).

Withdrawal

Goldstein and Volkow (2002) demonstrated that the relative cerebral blood flow values for the prefrontal cortex and the left lateral frontal cortex were significantly lower in the cocaine users (during an extended withdrawal state) than in the normal comparison subjects. They later showed in PET imaging studies of glucose metabolism decreases in regional brain glucose metabolism between cocaine abusers tested within two to four weeks of last cocaine use and cocaine abusers tested one week after last cocaine use (Volkow, 1991). During more protracted withdrawal (one to six weeks since last use), brain metabolism was found to be lower in cocaine abusers than in normal comparison subjects, an effect that was most accentuated in the frontal cortex (Volkow, 1992).

Studies of alcohol abusers have provided similar evidence. For example, lowered glucose metabolism was found in the frontal cortex in otherwise healthy alcoholic subjects with mean duration of alcohol withdrawal of eleven days (Volkow, 1992). In other studies, alcoholic subjects have shown less sensitivity to the lower metabolism induced by lorazepam, a benzodiazepine that facilitates GABA neurotransmission in the striatal-thalamo-orbitofrontal cortex circuit during early (one to four weeks) detoxification (Volkow, 1993) and in the orbitofrontal cortex during protracted (eight to eleven weeks) detoxification (Volkow, 1997), suggesting long-lasting drug-related adjustments in these brain regions. Persistent reduced glucose metabolism has also been demonstrated in the anterior cingulate cortex six to eight weeks after alcohol detoxification. Lower activity in the prefrontal cortex in alcoholic subjects during detoxification was also documented in other laboratories using slightly different study groups (Catafau, 1999). Alcoholic subjects show less metabolic activity in the striatum, thalamus and orbitofrontal cortex when exposed to the serotonin agonist m-chlorophenylpiperazine, reinforcing our understanding of the role of serotonin in alcoholism (Hommer, 1997).

Several studies from the laboratory of Dr. Volkow showed the role of dopamine in withdrawal. They documented in several studies of cocaine addicts early withdrawal (up to one month since last cocaine use), and protracted withdrawal (up to four months since last cocaine use), striatal dopamine response, and receptor availability were significantly lower than in normal comparison subjects (Volkow, 1997, 1990, 1993). Using PET imaging of a labeled dopamine agonist and glucose metabolism, Volkow also showed lower striatal dopamine D2 receptor binding in heroin, methamphetamine, and in alcoholic subjects (Wang, 1997; Volkow, 1996, 2001). The lower levels of striatal D2 receptors were found to be associated with lower metabolism in the orbitofrontal cortex and anterior cingulate gyrus in cocaine-addicted subjects and in the orbitofrontal cortex in methamphetamine abusers (Volkow, 1993, 2001).

In summary, withdrawal states are characterized by decreased metabolic function of multiple areas of the frontal lobe and striatum, areas critical to executive cognitive function and decision-making. Cognitive impairment due to addiction is addressed in detail in Chapter 6.

Primary Brain Regions <u>Deactivated</u> in Withdrawal and Damaged with Chronic Use

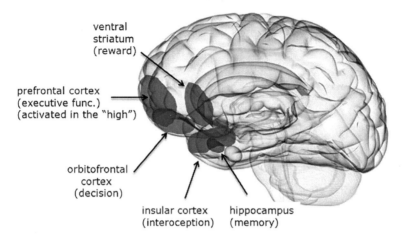

ventral striatum (reward)

prefrontal cortex (executive func.) (activated in the "high")

orbitofrontal cortex (decision)

insular cortex (interoception)

hippocampus (memory)

Chronic Changes

Everybody is aware that alcohol damages the brain. Doctors have observed atrophy in autopsy specimens, and early CT studies confirmed increased ventricular (central reservoirs of cerebral spinal fluid) and intrasulcal (spaces between the folds) volumes in alcoholics (Pfefferbaum, 1988). MRI studies have shown reduced volume in the frontal and temporal cortices, hippocampus, mammallary bodies and cerebellum, with greater loss seen in older age groups (Pfefferbaum, 1998). Reduced white matter in the temporal lobes has been related to a history of seizures, but it is not clear whether it is a cause or a consequence (Sullivan, 1996). MRI has also been valuable in examining changes in gross brain volume over time in alcoholics. Pfefferbaum (1995) showed an increase in frontal cortical grey matter volume in alcoholics abstinent for thirty days. These changes were initially attributed to "rehydration" but have also been attributed to sprouting of new dendrites and axons. MRI and proton MR spectroscopy (MRS) have provided clinicians with evidence that neuronal regeneration (as evidenced by increased axon metabolite, N-acetylaspartate/choline) is an important factor underlying the reversal of alcohol-induced atrophy (Bendszus, 2001).

Wernicke's encephalopathy and Korsakoff's syndrome are, respectively, acute and chronic clinical syndromes associated with thiamine deficiency seen in alcohol dependence. MRI studies in alcohol-dependent patients with these clinical features have identified widespread reductions in grey-matter volumes, especially in the thalamus, cerebellum, frontal and temporal regions, and medial and dorsal raphe nuclei. Significant shrinkage of mammallary bodies was seen in some non-amnesic alcoholics, but was universal in patients with Korsakoff's syndrome, suggesting a continuum of mammallary body pathology in chronic alcoholism (Sullivan, 1999). Classically, post-mortem work described greater gross damage to the white than grey matter from alcohol. A recent advance, diffusion tensor imaging (DTI), which shows subtle disruption of white matter tracts in the brain, has shown damage to the white matter in all brain regions, particularly in the genu and centrum semiovale, in alcoholics, in the absence of gross structural changes (Pfefferbaum, 2002).

Former alcoholics show reduced right anterior insula volumes that, notably, tend to increase with length of abstinence (Makris et al. 2008b). Similar reductions in insular volume and in cortical thickness have been reported for cocaine users (Franklin, 2002; Makris, 2008a). This might be anticipated given the high concentration within the insula of neurotransmitters, such as dopamine and opioids, that are highly relevant to the reinforcing and subjective effects of drugs of abuse (Baumgartner, 2006; Gaspar, 1989; Hurd, 2001). Structural changes within the insula are consistent with drug use impacting upon this area.

As might be expected, PET glucose metabolism and SPECT cerebral blood flow neuroimaging studies have shown reduced blood flow, perfusion or metabolism in individuals diagnosed with chronic alcohol dependence, with the frontal lobe being particularly compromised (Moselhy, 2001). *Improvement in cerebral activity is seen during early abstinence.* Volkow (1994) reported normalization of metabolism in the frontal lobes in abstinent alcoholics, as well as demonstrating that cerebral blood flow in the frontal lobes increases progressively with abstinence and returns to premorbid levels within four years (Gansler, 2000). George (1999) showed that alcoholics who underwent multiple detoxifications had advanced reduction in cerebral blood flow in the frontal lobes. Morphological changes identified with neuroimaging have been associated with neuropsychological impairment (Moselhy, 2001). A study in a healthy population of alcoholics found reduced medial-frontal lobe metabolism correlated with impairments in verbal fluency (Dao-Castellana, 1998).

MRI studies of structural changes in stimulant abusers have shown changes consistent with infarcts and hemorrhages, usually attributed to the vasoconstrictive properties of these drugs. Striatal hypertrophy has been reported in cocaine addicts, and is thought to be secondary to the depletion of dopamine and hypoperfusion (Jacobsen, 2001). Reduced levels of grey matter in several regions, including the orbitofrontal, cingulate, and temporal cortices, of cocaine addicts have been reported (Franklin, 2002). Diffusion tensor imaging has recently shown abnormalities in the white matter of the orbitofrontal cortex in cocaine addicts (Lim, 2002).

Cocaine addiction is associated with widespread reductions in metabolism and cerebral perfusion long after discontinued use (Kaufman, 1998; Volkow, 1988, Ernst, 2000). These findings are attributable to the vasoconstrictive effects of cocaine that result in cerebral infarcts (strokes). A similar pattern is seen with amphetamine abuse (Wolkin, 1987; de Wit, 1991). Methamphetamine abuse is also associated with reduced cerebral metabolic activity, particular in the striatum, together with hypermetabolism in parietal cortex, which is thought to reflect gliosis/ inflammation (Volkow, 1991; Chang, 2002). As with alcoholism, increased cerebral blood flow and metabolism during the early withdrawal period from cocaine have been reported in the orbitofrontal cortex followed by hypometabolism (Ernst, 2000). It is likely that this initial increase in metabolism is secondary to craving, which is high in early abstinence. Volkow hypothesized that reduced activity in the orbitofrontal cortex was a result of reduced dopaminergic input, since activity here correlated with striatal DRD2 levels (Volkow, 1999). Increasing dopaminergic activity with methylphenidate did not increase metabolism in the orbitofrontal cortex of all cocaine addicts, but in those that it was, craving was experienced. This study suggests that increasing dopaminergic function is not sufficient to reverse damage from cocaine and that the orbitofrontal cortex is critical to craving.

Functional MRI has been used to examine the effects of drug abuse on cognitive processes thought to be impaired by, or involved in drug abuse. Using functional MRI researchers have found that methamphetamine dependence was associated with reduced activation in the prefrontal cortex reflected as impaired decision-making, and that decreased activation in the OFC correlated with the duration of methamphetamine abuse (Paulus,

2002). Given the evidence of frontal lobe and insular dysfunction in addicts, compromise on the cognitive processes is predicted. This subject is covered in detail in Chapter 6.

Summary of Imaging Studies

To summarize, during drug craving there are predominant activations in the frontal lobe—inclusive of the orbitofrontal cortex and anterior cingulate cortex—and temporal lobe insula. During acute intoxication, the majority of the studies show activation in the prefrontal cortex and anterior cingulate gyrus when using either the cerebral blood flow or functional MRI oxygen utilization methods. Prefrontal activation appears to be associated with the subjective perception of intoxication, the reinforcing effects of the drug, or enhanced mood.

Withdrawal states are characterized by decreased metabolic function of multiple areas of the frontal lobe and striatum, areas critical to executive cognitive function and decision-making. Chronic injury is drug specific, although predominantly in the frontal lobe and insula with the majority of drugs studied.

Clark A.: Phenomenon of Craving, After 21 Years Sober

Clark is a friend from my home AA group. He has been sober for twenty-one years. He is in his sixties, intelligent, friendly, and came to the meeting once or twice a week for many years. Before he came to AA, he was drinking a fifth of vodka every day. Trouble with his wife brought him to the rooms of Alcoholics Anonymous. He looked like he was working a good program of sobriety.

When my group did not see him for a month or so, we thought he was on vacation. We found out later that Clark had relapsed. AA friends performed a twelfth-step call to his home. They found him a wreck. He was disheveled and drunk. He picked up a drink because his wife of over thirty years was dying of cancer. Between the grief and fear of loneliness, he was distraught. To ease his distress, he took the idea of "tying one on" only for a day. Once he had a couple of cocktails, the phenomenon of craving took grip, and soon he was falling-down drunk. Within a week of having his first drink in twenty-one years, his tolerance returned and he was drinking a fifth of vodka a day again.

Clark's story is very common and referred to frequently in the text and stories in the *Big Book of AA*. The neuroadaptations induced in his brain through drinking, twenty-one years ago, were still present today. He can *never* drink like a nonalcoholic again. His AA friends stayed with Clark through his withdrawals and got him back on track in the program of AA. He is still sober today, one year later.

Chapter 5

Stress and Addiction: Like Gasoline and Fire

Paul H.: All Stressed Out

Paul H. is a well-respected attorney with a busy practice in New York City. He is also a recovering alcoholic who, after five years of sobriety, picked up "just one" drink to sooth some mental distress over workplace politics. After one drink, he had several more and was completely intoxicated in a few hours. In the swell of his morning hangover, he swore to stop. After two years of occasional, sporadic drinking and drunkenness, the talons of his alcoholism gripped stronger and stronger, and he began drinking every day, sometimes very heavily. Recognizing changes in his appearance and behavior, his employer and wife intervened on him, demanding he go to inpatient, residential treatment.

After ninety days of treatment and abstinence, Paul went home on an authorized pass. While at home, he was exposed to acute familial and occupational stress. Six weeks sober, Paul's stress level spiked, he was extremely "uncomfortable," and, without accessing available, alternative coping mechanisms, he drank. He told me, at that very moment, he was at the point that he couldn't live with alcohol and he couldn't live without it. He said he "was all stressed out." He returned to the treatment center to continue his recovery, desperate to find a solution to his malady. Today, Paul is three years sober.

Stress and Reward Systems Intimately Linked

The notion that stress leads to drug abuse in vulnerable individuals and relapse in addicts is not new. My personal experience and several theoretical models of addiction have proposed that *stress* increases risk of drug abuse and relapse. Vast clinical observations suggest that exposure to stress can initiate or increase drug use and is associated with craving and relapse in addicts.

Brain neuro-endocrine (neural-hormonal) stress systems are intimately related to the reward system described in previous chapters. The center of endocrine function, the hypothalamic-pituitary axis, has direct neural connection with reward circuits, and secreted hormones modify the neural functions of these circuits. "Stress and addiction" are like "gasoline and fire."

Current trends in addiction literature suggest that changes in brain stress systems alter the ability of addicts to cope with stress, particularly with respect to perpetuation of addictive behaviors and relapse. *It is uniformly accepted by addiction professionals that stress perpetuates addiction in as much as modifications in the brain reward systems themselves.* There has been a dramatic increase in research to understand the neuroendocrine circuits associated with stress and those underlying addictive behaviors. Several animal laboratory studies have shown that stress exposure enhances drug self-administration. Furthermore, recent brain imaging and endocrine studies in humans have shown neuroadaptations in brain stress circuits due to chronic drug addiction.

Stress: Definitions

The term *"stress"* obtained its contemporary connotations in the early twentieth century. It was first employed in a biological context by the endocrinologist Dr. Hans Selye in the 1930s. It is a form of the Middle English *destresse*, derived from the Latin *stringere*, "to draw (the string) tight." As used by Dr. Selye, it refers to the general state of an organism exposed to physical or emotional threats, actual or imagined. In 1975, Dr. Selye further elaborated his "stress model" to describe *eustress* (good stress) and *distress* (bad stress). *Eustress* refers to the condition in which stress, physical or mental, enhances function, such as muscular strength training or mentally challenging work. *Distress* refers to persistent stress that is not resolved through coping or adaptation, which may lead to a physical or mental pathologic state or injury.

In psychology, the term "stress" includes any process involving perception, interpretation, response, and adaptation to harmful, threatening, or challenging events (Lazarus, 1984). *Stress* covers a wide range of phenomena, from mild irritation to drastic biological dysfunction, even death. Lazarus, a psychologist, argued that cognitive processes of appraisal are central in determining whether a situation is potentially threatening, and both personal and environmental factors influence this primary appraisal, which then triggers the stress response and influences the selection of coping processes.

In clarifying the term "stress" and its components, it is important to note that while stress is often associated with negative affect and distress, it includes states that may be perceived as pleasant and exciting (Selye, 1976). For example, mild, brief or controllable "challenge states" perceived as exciting simultaneously activate brain stress and reward circuits and, therefore, are perceived as pleasurable. These responses are fundamental to biological and cognitive adaptation and learning (Hennessey, 1979). The "stress" one feels in anticipation of sex or winning the lottery, riding a roller coaster, parachuting, or fast skiing, is an example. The anticipatory state of these activities can be quite addictive in and of itself.

The reward and stress circuits are also intimately related to our the brain's memory and learning centers, an evolutionarily adaptive feature of our neuroanatomy: We learn to fear that which will harm us; we have to learn to fear to survive! However, more severe stress is associated with states of increased intensity of affect, greater uncontrollability and unpredictability, and greater danger, resulting in increased magnitude of the stress response and *discomfort* (Frankenhauser 1980; Lovallo, 1997). Thus, the dimensions of intensity, controllability, and predictability are important in understanding the role of stress in maladaptive responses, such as chronic anxiety, depression, harmful addictive behaviors, drug abuse and addiction.

Acute vs. Chronic, Adaptive vs. Maladaptive Stress

The acute stress response, also called the *"fight-or-flight"* response was first described by biologist Walter Cannon in the 1920's as a theory that animals react to threats with a general discharge of the sympathetic (stimulatory) nerves of the autonomic nervous system. The response was later recognized as the first stage of a general adaptation syndrome that regulates stress responses among vertebrates and other phylogenetically higher organisms. The autonomic nervous system provides the rapid response to stress, engaging the sympathetic nervous system and withdrawing the parasympathetic (inhibitory) nervous system, thereby enacting accelerated cardiovascular, respiratory, musculoskeletal, and metabolic responses. The stress response begins in the brain with sympathetic nervous discharges and is enhanced by the adrenal glands (endocrine glands), located above the kidneys, with release of epinephrine and norepinephrine (catecholamines, a.k.a. adrenaline). The adrenal release is triggered by neurotransmitters released from nerves arising in the brainstem targeting the glands.

Brain and adrenal catecholamines, stimulatory synaptic transmitters, and circulatory hormones facilitate immediate physical reactions serving as a rapid-acting global alarm system. Catecholamines trigger increases in heart rate and contractility, increased breathing, dilation of blood vessels in the muscles while constricting blood vessels in the gut, slowing digestion, liberation of glucose and fat for muscular action, acceleration of reflexes, tightening skeletal muscles, relaxation of sphincters, and tunnel vision. A surge of catecholamines affects the brain by activating innate spontaneous behaviors necessary to combat or escape.

Specifically, in response to acute stress, a collection of neurons in the brainstem known as the *locus coeruleus* and cells in the adrenal medulla (center of the adrenal gland), collectively known as the locus-coeruleus/ neuro-endocrine (LC/NE) system, are acutely activated and use brain locus ceruleus epinephrine to execute autonomic and neuroendocrine responses. Normally, when a person is in a serene, non-stimulated state, the "firing" of neurons in the locus ceruleus is minimal. A novel stimulus, once perceived, is relayed from the sensory cortex of the brain through the thalamus and limbic system (especially the amygdala) to the brainstem. This signaling route increases the rate of adrenergic activity in the locus ceruleus, and the person becomes alert and attentive to the environment. If a stimulus is perceived as a threat, a more intense and prolonged discharge of the locus ceruleus activates the sympathetic (stimulatory) division of the autonomic nervous system as well as the hypothalamic-pituitary-adrenal axis (HPA axis).

The HPA axis constitutes the neuro-endocrine (neuro-hormonal) system involved in the fight-or-flight response. It involves interactions between the hypothalamus, the pituitary gland, and the adrenal glands. In response to a perceived stressor, neurons with cell bodies in the periventricular nuclei (PVN) of the hypothalamus secrete corticotropin-releasing factor (CRF) and arginine-vasopressin (AVP) into the pituitary gland. This results in release of adrenocorticotropic hormone (ACTH) from the pituitary into the general bloodstream, which results in secretion of *cortisol* and other glucocorticoids (glucose-forming hormones) from the adrenal cortex (outer layer). These circulating corticoids, particularly cortisol, engage the entire body in the organism's response to stress and ultimately contribute to the termination of the response via inhibitory feedback on the hypothalamus.

Acute or chronic stress, through sympathetic (stimulatory) nervous system arousal, inhibits functions that are controlled by the parasympathetic (inhibitory) nervous system. In this manner, the stress response halts or slows down "non-essential" functions, such as sexual responses and the digestive system, to focus the body's fight-or-flight resources on the stressor situation, adaptive in evolutionary terms. In modern environments, more protracted, chronic stress typically causes negative, maladaptive effects like constipation, anorexia, erectile dysfunction, difficulty urinating, and difficulty maintaining sexual arousal. Stress-induced shutting down of the reproductive system increases the risk of miscarriage.

Stress Response

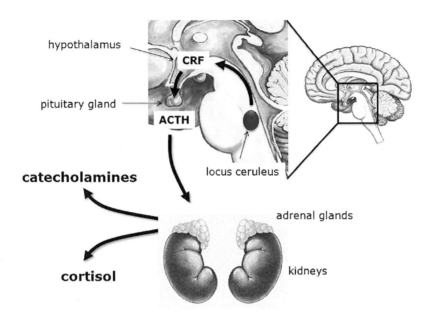

Cortisol is the major stress hormone and can show chronic elevations in response to protracted stress. Cortisol's primary function is to increase blood sugar through gluconeogenesis. Gluconeogenesis literally means "making sugar" and involves the breakdown of protein and fat to provide metabolites that can be converted to glucose in the liver. The process of gluconeogenesis aids in fat, protein, and carbohydrate metabolism. Cortisol also serves to reduce inflammation through suppressing the immune system. (Related hormones, cortisone and hydrocortisone, are frequently used as a key anti-inflammatory component in drugs that treat skin rashes, in nasal sprays that treat sinusitis and in inhalers for asthma.) Cortisol is released in response to stress and low levels of blood glucose or glucocorticoids (a class of hormones inclusive of cortisol and less prevalent, but related hormones). In short bursts, therefore, cortisol is quite advantageous and evolutionarily adaptive for survival.

In response to protracted stress, cortisol can be chronically elevated, leading to adverse physical and mental effects, an evolutionarily maladaptive state. Cortisol counteracts insulin and inhibits the peripheral utilization of glucose (insulin resistance) by impeding insulin-sensitive glucose transporters in the cell membrane. In insulin-resistant individuals, insulin becomes less effective at lowering blood sugars. The resulting increase in blood glucose may raise levels outside the normal range and cause adverse health effects, as seen in type 2 diabetes. Although there is a short boost of the immune system in response to acute stress (perhaps due to an ancient need to fight the inflammation and infection in wounds received during interaction with a predator), prolonged stress responses result in chronic suppression of the immune system, leaving the body open to infections. Chronically elevated cortisol causes excessive collagen breakdown in skin, muscle, and bone, leading to skin thinning, muscular wasting and osteoporosis. Chronically elevated cortisol leads to excessive abdominal fat deposition in the abdomen (mid-abdominal obesity). Cortisol causes excess gastric acid secretion and ulcer formation, and excessive sodium and fluid retention (bloating).

Chronic stress can also cause memory impairment and hippocampal atrophy through the action of cortisol on this brain nucleus, likely through glucose starvation (Bremner, 1995, 1997). Similar atrophy can be seen in the brain's frontal lobes in response to chronic stress (Carrion, 2001). Finally, via cortisol, chronic stress increases blood pressure by increasing the sensitivity of arteries to epinephrine and norepinephrine (in the absence of cortisol, there is widespread dilation of arteries). Cortisol-mediated vasoconstriction can accelerate atherosclerosis and lead to heart attacks and strokes.

Emotional Distress: Appraisal, Coping, and Learning

General emotion expressions of stress include fear, anxiety, anger, excitement, pleasure, and sadness. Examples of emotional stressors include interpersonal conflict, loss of a relationship, death of a close family member, and loss of a child. Signs of emotional distress may be cognitive, emotional, physical, or behavioral. Signs include poor judgment; a general negative outlook; excessive worrying; moodiness; irritability; agitation; inability to relax; feeling lonely, isolated, or depressed; aches and pains; diarrhea or constipation; nausea; dizziness; chest pain; rapid heartbeat; eating too much or not enough; sleeping too much or not enough; social withdrawal; procrastination or neglect of responsibilities; nervous habits, such as pacing about and nail biting; neck and back pains; and increased alcohol, nicotine, or drug consumption.

In general, emotional distress causes mental and physical *discomfort* in the individual and a perturbation in cognitive, affective, and physiological homeostasis (Carver, 1999). The discomfort of emotional distress motivates individuals to adapt, to reduce stress by using coping strategies. The goal of coping strategies is to return to a *comfortable* state, to regain homeostasis. Given that difficulties in maintaining homeostasis have been conceptualized as central to addiction (Koob, 1997), a closer look at stress-related coping and its neural representations is warranted.

Stress reactions depend on the specific features of the stressful situation, a cognitive and emotional *appraisal* of the event, including prior emotional state of the individual and available coping resources. Perception of a threat or challenge first relies on brain information processing circuits, such as the primary sensory projections and sensory association cortices of the frontal, parietal, and occipital lobes (McEwen, 1993). Attention circuits are activated in the anterior cingulate cortex. Cognitive appraisal relies on internal cognitive processes, primarily in the frontal lobe. Affective (emotional) appraisal occurs in the limbic structures and perilimbic cortices, such as the temporal lobe insula, a process called *interoception.* The limbic-affective processing circuits, particularly the amygdala, interact with the frontal lobe, particularly the orbitofrontal and medial pre-frontal cortices, to determine the meaning and significance of events.

Frontal and temporal lobes, limbic structures and perilimbic cortices are intimately connected with the dopaminergic reward system to play a key role in the learning of adaptive approaches or avoidance responses and the mediation of goal-directed behaviors, functions that are important in the development of cognitive and affective coping (Gaffan, 1993; Robbins, 1996; Lovallo, 1997). In addition to release of mesolimbic dopamine, brain catecholamines in other limbic regions and endogenous opiates contribute to enhance adaptation to stress. Furthermore, the serotonin, acetylcholine, and GABA systems are also involved, although to a lesser extent, in modulating brain CRF and cortisol production, as well as sympathetic nervous system circuits (Arborelius, 1999).

In simple terms, when stressed, in fight-or-flight terminology, one can either change the stressor (fight it), avoid the stressor (take flight), or change the perception or appraisal of the stressor through cognitive and affective coping strategies, including mood-altering substances. As addressed in earlier chapters, many animal species and ancient man used mood-altering substances to create a sense of false Darwinian fitness. The psychology literature elaborates on these basic coping mechanisms: *Cognitive coping* involves cognitive and behavioral strategies—such as cognitive restructuring, planning and preparation for recurrence of the event—consideration of alternate options, and behavioral modifications involving direct action aimed at altering the source of stress or one's relationship to it. *Affective coping* is the management of one's emotional distress associated with the stressful event rather than the cause of the stress. *Avoidance coping* is aimed at avoiding any acknowledgment of the event or giving up the attempt to do anything about the event (Lazarus 1966; Lazarus and Folkman 1984; Carver et al. 1989).

Cognitive, affective, and avoidance coping strategies can employ mind—and mood-altering substances. In this context, drug use can be temporarily adaptive in that it relieves the discomfort of stress. Drug use, however, is mostly maladaptive: Alterations in sensory perception, loss of motor coordination, and poor decision-making can lead to a multitude of negative consequences, including death.

Observations of Stress-Related Drug Abuse in Humans

Numerous human studies have reported a positive association between stresses associated with adverse life events, chronic emotional and physical distress, and increased drug abuse. Individuals with early physical and sexual abuse histories are at risk to abuse substances and report an earlier age of onset of substance abuse (Demboet, 1988; Harrison, 1997; Widom, 1999). Alcohol consumption is positively associated with high stress levels, lack of social support and avoidance coping (Aro, 1981; Cronkit, 1984; DeFrank, 1987; Chassin, 1988; Pohorecky, 1991). Furthermore, drinking and drug use as a coping response to stress is positively associated with dependence symptoms and compulsive drug use, while drug use for social and enhancement reasons is not associated with problematic levels of use (Cooper, 1992; Laurent, 1997).

Studies in adolescents show that higher levels of stress and maladaptive coping, along with low parental support, predict escalation of nicotine, alcohol and marijuana use (Kaplan, 1986; Newcomb, 1988; Kaplan, 1992; Wills, 1996). Anxiety and mood disorders and behavioral conduct problems in adolescents are associated with an increased frequency and regular use of substances, such as alcohol, nicotine and marijuana (King, 1996; Rohde, 1996; Kandel, 1997; Riggs, 1999; Rao, 1999). Increased frequency of substance abuse is more likely to follow the occurrence of behavior problems and psychiatric disorders in adolescents (Kessler, 1996; Rohde, 1996; Riggs, 1999).

Psychiatric illness and substance use disorders are highly associated in adults as well, with lifetime prevalence rates above 50 percent for co-occurrence of any psychiatric disorder with substance abuse (Regieret, 1990; Kessler, 1994, 1996). Several studies have shown a significant association between prevalence of mood and anxiety disorders, including post-traumatic stress disorder (PTSD), behavioral conduct problems, and increased risk of substance use disorders (Kandel, 1997; King, 1996; Riggs, 1999; Sinha, 2002; Kessler, 1996; Brady, 2005).

Two recent studies have examined lifetime exposure to stressors and the impact of cumulative stress on addiction vulnerability after accounting for a number of control factors, such as race/ethnicity, gender, socioeconomic status, prior drug abuse, prevalence of psychiatric disorders, family history of substance use, and behavioral and conduct problems (Turner, 2003; Lloyd, 2008). Cumulative adversity or stress was assessed using a checklist method and by counting the number of different events that were experienced in a given period during the life span. The types of adverse events significantly associated with addiction vulnerability were parental divorce or conflict; abandonment; being forced to live apart from parents; loss of a child by death or removal; unfaithfulness of a significant other; loss of home to natural disaster; death of a loved one; emotional abuse or neglect; sexual abuse; rape; physical abuse by a parent, caretaker, family member, spouse, or significant other; being victim of a shooting or other violent acts; and observing violent victimization. These represent highly stressful and emotionally distressing events, which are typically uncontrollable and unpredictable in nature. The effects of distal (events occurring more than one year prior) and proximal stress experiences (events during the most recent one-year period), and their effects on meeting criteria for substance use disorders, were assessed. Both studies indicate that the cumulative number of stressful events was predictive of alcohol and drug dependence in a dose-dependent manner. Both distal and proximal events significantly and independently affected addiction vulnerability. Furthermore, the dose-dependent effects of cumulative stressors on risk for addiction existed for both genders and for Caucasian, African American, and Hispanic race/ethnic groups.

Human laboratory studies have shown increased drug taking after stressful, as opposed to non-stressful, situations. In a study of social drinkers, exposure to stressors, such as fear of interpersonal evaluation, anger due to provocation by a confederate, and failure feedback on exposure to insolvable problems, led to increased alcohol consumption as compared with drinking behavior in non-stressful situations (Higgins, 1975; Marlatt, 1975; Hull, 1983). Alcoholics, as compared with non-alcoholics, are also known to increase alcohol intake in response to stressful situations (Miller, 1974). In smokers, smoking increases after exposure to high anxiety, as compared with low anxiety-provoking situations (Pomerleau, 1987). These findings indicate that in social drinkers, smokers and alcoholics, stress exposure enhances drug self-administration, likely in an effort to cope with stress.

Animal Studies of Stress-Induce Drug Use

Evidence from animal studies has shown that specific types of stressful experiences in early life may increase the vulnerability to drug use. In a series of studies, Higley and colleagues (1991, 1993) studied alcohol consumption behavior in rhesus monkeys reared by mothers (normal condition) or by peers (stressed condition) for the first six months of their life. As adults, peer-reared monkeys consumed significantly more amounts of alcohol than mother-reared monkeys. Furthermore, when stress was increased in the adult monkeys by social separation, mother-reared monkeys increased their levels of alcohol consumption to that of peer-reared monkeys, while peer-reared monkeys maintained their level of alcohol consumption. Similarly, in studies of rodent populations, social separation or isolation in early life, in contrast to group housing, has been shown to increase self-administration of morphine and cocaine (Adler, 1975; Kostowski, 1977; Alexander, 1978; Schenk, 1987). A study by Kosten and colleagues (2000) showed that isolation as neonates in adult rats enhances acquisition of cocaine self-administration as adults. These studies suggest that stress in early and adult life both appear to increase self-administration of drugs and alcohol.

Further research has found that chronically stressed infant monkeys have increased levels of CRF in their cerebrospinal fluid (CSF) (Coplan, 1996). Such hypersensitivity of the CRF-HPA system has been linked to chronic distress states, such as anxiety and mood disorders (Arborelius, 1999). Sapolsky and colleagues (1997) reported that chronic social stress associated with social subordination in wild baboons is associated with hypercortisolism (chronically elevated cortisol), a state commonly found among individuals with depressive symptoms and anxiety disorders. In a series of studies, Meaney and colleagues found long-lasting changes in the CRF-HPA stress response in rodents exposed to stress as neonates. (Meaney, 1993; Plotsky, 1993). In these rodents, they observed increased sensitivity to stressors and an altered HPA response and behavioral stress response throughout development and adult life (Meaney, 1993).

Other studies have shown that rats with high reactivity to novel situations, as measured by high circulating cortisol levels, are at increased vulnerability to self-administration of psycho-stimulants, such as amphetamines (Piazza, 1989, 1996). Fahlke (2000) showed that primates stressed early in life and demonstrating elevated cortisol levels at that time self-administer alcohol in excess as adults, compared with non-stressed animals. Therefore, differences in response to stressful events and previous experience of stressful events appear to predispose animals to an increased vulnerability to self-administer addictive substances. It has been proposed by these authors that drug-and alcohol-use vulnerability may be linked to hyper-responsiveness of the CRF-HPA system to stress.

Several studies in adult animals have shown that acute exposure to stress increases initiation and escalation of drug use and abuse (Sinha, 2001, 2005). In rodent models, stress can be in the form of a tail pinch, foot shock, social defeat, social isolation, restraint, or novel environment. Researchers observed some variation in drug usage secondary to stressor type, genetic background of animals, and variations by drug type (Lu, 2005; Cleck, 2008). A study by Piazza (1991) is particularly interesting: Rats that showed increased agitation and locomotor activity and high cortisol levels upon exposure to a novel environment were termed "high responders" (showing elevated stress), whereas "low responders" exhibited decreased locomotor activity and lower cortisol levels (low stress). Following this initial classification, animals were trained to self-administer cocaine. Low responders did not learn to self administer cocaine, whereas robust self-administration was observed in rats assessed as high responders. The most interesting aspect of Piazza's study was his second experiment: daily cortisol administration induced and maintained amphetamine self-administration in the low-responding rats, effectively switching their behavior, and accelerated cocaine self-administration, to that of high responders.

Elimination of the cortisol response by adrenalectomy, by treatment with metyrapone, a cortisol synthesis blocker, or by ketoconazole, a cortisol receptor blocker, decreases stress-induced stimulant self-administration in rodents (Goeders, 1996; Piazza, 1996; Mantsch, 1999), and alcohol consumption in high alcohol-preferring rodents (Fahlke, 1994, 2000). These studies support the hypothesis that a hyper-responsive HPA axis leading to increased circulating cortisol and its stimulation of dopaminergic transmission in mesolimbic pathways appears to enhance drug self-administration.

Neurobiology of Stress and Drug Addiction

It has been postulated that psychiatric disorders, such as anxiety and affective disorders, are manifestations of chronic stress states that are associated with dysregulated brain stress circuits (Plotsky, 1995; Arborelius, 1999). Adaptations in brain stress circuits may lead to a greater sensitivity to the reinforcing properties of mood-altering drugs, thereby increasing the frequency of drug use and addiction in these individuals. Depression and anxiety are chronic stress states associated with hypercortisolism (Plotsky, 1995; Arborelius, 1999). It is hypothesized that high levels of circulating cortisol may mediate increased drug self-administration in individuals with these disorders who also have a vulnerability to drug abuse. Altered cortisol levels have been linked to many psychiatric syndromes, including affective disorders and PTSD (Chrousos, 1992; Nemeroff, 2000). Some studies have also suggested that increased brain CRF and noradrenergic (norepinephrine and epinephrine) activation, more than elevated cortisol levels, mediates stress-induced drug seeking and relapse (Shaham, 1997, 1998; Erb, 1998; Stewart, 2000).

The aforementioned studies have shown that the stress response facilitates drug self-administration. Further studies have shown that activation of brain stress circuits increases dopaminergic neurotransmission in brain reward mesolimbic circuits (Dunn, 1988; Kalivas, 1989; Prasad, 1995; Piazza, 1996). Increased dopaminergic transmission in these pathways is critical for the reinforcing properties of abusive drugs. Thus, stress co-activates brain stress circuits and the putative reward circuitry simultaneously, thereby providing a common neural substrate by which stress may enhance the drug-taking experience and increase drug self-administration.

Most major theories of addiction postulate that acute and chronic stress play an important role in the motivation to abuse addictive substances (Russell, 1975; Leventhal, 1980; Shiffman 1982; Marlatt, 1985; Wills,

1985; Koob, 1997). The popular *tension reduction* (Conger, 1956; Sher, 1982) and *self-medication models* (Khantzian, 1985) have proposed that people use drugs to enhance mood and alleviate emotional distress. The *stress-coping model* of addiction proposes that use of addictive substances serves to both reduce negative affect and increase positive affect, thereby reinforcing drug taking as an effective, albeit maladaptive, coping strategy (Shiffman 1982; Wills, 1985). Marlatt's *relapse prevention model* (Marlatt, 1985) states that in addition to other bio-psychosocial risk factors such as parental substance use, peer pressure, and positive expectancies over the potential benefits of using substances, individuals with poor coping resources are at increased risk for addiction.

These models are based on the assumption that the motivation to enhance mood is greater in acute and chronic stress states. *Initially a drug may be used to modulate tension or distress. Subsequently, with repeated administration, it may become a ubiquitous response for both stress relief and mood enhancement: addiction engages.* Motivations to relieve stress (negative reinforcement) or mood enhancement (positive reinforcement) can act synergistically to increase the vulnerability to drug addiction. Based on their observations, notable addiction researchers, Koob and Le Moal (1997) have proposed a biological model that links the negative and positive reinforcement aspects of drug use. They postulate that stress leads to state-related changes in brain reward circuits, resulting in a greater sensitivity to the reinforcing properties of drugs and thereby increasing the motivation to use drugs compulsively. Thus, stress appears to "prime" brain reward systems, thereby enhancing the reinforcing efficacy of drugs, particularly in those vulnerable to addiction (Piazza and Le Moal, 1998). This neurobiological model provides an explanation for how the transition from experimental drug use as a coping mechanism to addiction may occur, particularly in the genetically vulnerable.

Most commonly abused drugs that stimulate brain reward pathways (dopaminergic systems)—such as alcohol, nicotine, cocaine, amphetamines, opiates, and marijuana—activate brain stress systems (Baumann 1995; Heesch 1995; Kreek, 1998). These drugs induce chronic, if not permanent, neuroadaptations in reward circuits inclusive of increased number and strength of neural connections. As stated earlier, several studies have shown that activation of brain stress circuits increases dopaminergic neurotransmission in the nucleus accumbens and other reward pathways, the initiating event for further neuroadaptations (Thierry, 1976; Dunn,

1988; Kalivas, 1989; Prasad, 1995; Piazza, 1996; Goeders, 1997). Several studies have also shown that stress and concomitant increases in CRF and cortisol enhance glutamate activity in the ventral tegmental area (VTA), which in turn enhances dopamine production (Saal, 2003; Ungless, 2003; Wang, 2005). Suppression of cortisol by adrenalectomy reduces levels of dopamine in the reward nucleus accumbens and in responses to stress and psychostimulants (Piazza 1996; Barrot 2000). Human brain imaging studies have further shown that stress-related increases in cortisol are associated with dopamine accumulation in the ventral striatum (VS) (Takahashi, 1998; Oswald, 2005).

In addition to a role in reward, human imaging studies and other data have shown that the VS is also involved in aversive conditioning, the experience of aversive, negative, or pain stimuli, as well as the anticipation of such stimuli (Sorg, 1991; Becerra, 2001; Jensen, 2003). These studies indicate a role for the mesolimbic dopamine pathways beyond reward processing, one that more broadly involves motivation and attention to any salient (aversive/bad or appetitive/good) events, and this response is critical to learning. An organism, animal or human, must learn to avoid aversive or threatening circumstances as much as it needs to learn to be directed toward rewarding circumstances. An organism must learn to fear to survive. Psychologists believe this adaptive learning response to aversive stimuli accounts for humans' "addiction" to roller-coaster rides and horror movies.

Stress Hormones in Tolerance and Withdrawal States

It is well-known that chronic abuse of addictive substances results in hallmark symptoms of dependence, compulsive drug use, tolerance, and withdrawal. Studies have shown that tolerance and withdrawal are associated with alterations in brain stress circuits, namely the HPA axis and autonomic sympathetic nervous system. During active drug use, alcoholics, chronic smokers, and cocaine addicts show hypercortisolism (Wilkins, 1982; Wand, 1991; Mello, 1997), whereas opiate addicts show reduced cortisol levels (Ho, 1977; Facchinetti, 1985). Acute withdrawal states from opiates, alcohol, and cocaine are associated with increases in CRF levels in CSF, plasma ACTH, cortisol, and catecholamine levels (Adinoff, 1990, 1991; Vescovi, 1992; Ehrenreich, 1997; Tsuda, 1996; Mello, 1997; Kreek, 1998). Early abstinence states are associated with a blunted HPA axis hormone response in alcoholics, while hyper-responsiveness of HPA axis hormones in response to metyrapone (drug that blocks cortisol synthesis) has been reported in opiate and cocaine addicts (Kreek 1997; Schluger 1998). Others studies have showed tolerance in the HPA axis response to cocaine, alcohol, nicotine, and opiates with chronic abuse (Eisenman 1969; Delitala 1983; Friedman 1987; Mendelson 1998). These findings suggest that active drug use, acute and protracted withdrawal, and tolerance symptoms are associated with alterations in brain stress circuits.

Early abstinence from alcohol, cocaine, opiates, nicotine, and marijuana leads to irritability, anxiety, emotional distress, sleep problems, dysphoria, aggressive behaviors, and extreme drug craving. The severity of the withdrawal symptoms is known to predict treatment outcome and relapse rates. In general, studies have shown that the greater the dependence, the greater the withdrawal severity, and the greater the susceptibility to poor treatment outcome and relapse (McLellan 1983; Carroll 1993; Doherty 1995; Tennant 1991; Mulvaney 1999).

Withdrawal is a biological and psychological *distressed* state associated with neuroadaptive changes in brain stress and reward circuits (Koob, 1997; Kreek, 1998; Volkow, 2000). Several studies have shown that acute withdrawal states are associated with increases in CRF levels in CSF, plasma ACTH, cortisol, and catecholamine levels (Koob, 1997, Mello, 1997; Kreek, 1998). Early abstinence is associated with high basal cortisol responses and a blunted or suppressed ACTH and cortisol response to pharmacological and psychological challenges in alcoholics and chronic smokers, while hyper-responsiveness of the HPA axis has been reported in opiate and cocaine addicts (Kreek, 1997). Furthermore, withdrawal and abstinence from chronic alcohol is also associated with altered sympathetic and parasympathetic responses (Ingjaldsson, 2003; Ramussen, 2006; Rechlin, 1996; Sinha, 2008). These studies emphasize the profound effects of drug use and abuse on physiological stress responses. In addition, as discussed in the previous chapter, although acute administration of drugs increases mesolimbic dopamine, regular and chronic use of addictive drugs leads to withdrawal states with down-regulated mesolimbic dopamine as well as noradrenergic pathways.

Effects of Stress on Drug Craving

Drug craving, or physiological *"wanting,"* is a prominent feature of addiction. Some have called it a *"fleshy hunger."* Negative affective states, stress or withdrawal-related distress have also been associated with increases in drug craving (Childress, 1994; Cooney, 1997; Sinha, 1999a, 2000a). In particular, craving and compulsive seeking are invoked strongly with stress exposure, which can become a potent trigger for relapse. Although external cues produce craving and reactivity in the laboratory, presence of negative affect, stress, and abstinence symptomatology has been predictive of relapse in community environments (Killen, 1997; Doherty, 1996; Cooney, 1997). Most researchers agree that heightened craving or wanting of a drug is the behavioral manifestation of molecular and cellular changes in the stress and dopamine pathways discussed previously.

Dr. Talih Sinha of the Yale University School of Medicine has widely studied the effects of stress on drug cravings. In one of his groups studies, drug craving and stress responses were assessed in abstinent addicts in residential treatment. They exposed these abstinent addicts to stressful and non-stressful drug visual cues and neutral, relaxing visual cues (Sinha, 2003). This group found that, in cocaine-addicted individuals, stress imagery elicited emotions of fear, sadness, and anger as compared with the stress of public speaking, which elicited increases in fear but not anger or sadness. In addition, imagery of personal stressors produced significant increases in cocaine craving, while public speaking did not (Sinha, 2000). They observed significant increases in heart rate, salivary cortisol, drug craving, and subjective anxiety with imagery exposure to stress cues and non-stress drug cues as compared with neutral relaxing cues in cocaine-dependent individuals. In additional studies, this research group has shown that both stress and alcohol-related cues similarly increase craving, anxiety, negative emotions, and physiological responses in abstinent alcoholics (Fox, 2007). On the other hand, recently abstinent alcoholics showed a suppressed HPA cortisol response to stress compared with non-addicted counterparts. Similarly, both stress and drug-related cues increased craving in naltrexone-treated (naltrexone is an opiate blocker), opiate-addicted individuals (Hyman, 2007).

In addition to altered HPA cortisol responses, Sinha's group found increases in catecholamines (norepinephrine and epinephrine) in a study of the effect of stress on abstinent cocaine addicts (Sinha, 2003). Furthermore, in this study they found that levels of catecholamines remain elevated for over an hour after the experiment. In another study, Sinha compared abstinent cocaine-dependent individuals with a demographically matched group of healthy social drinkers, using individually calibrated emotional stress and drug/alcohol cue-related imagery compared with neutral imagery. In this study, they found that cocaine-dependent individuals showed enhanced sensitivity to emotional distress and physiological arousal and higher levels of drug craving to both stress and drug-cue exposure compared with controls (Fox, 2008).

In a similar study, comparing four-week abstinent alcoholics to matched social drinkers, Sinha's group found that recovering alcoholics at four weeks abstinent showed greater levels of basal heart rate and salivary cortisol levels compared with control drinkers. Upon stress and alcohol-cue exposure, they showed persistently greater subjective distress, alcohol craving, and blood pressure responses but a suppressed heart rate and cortisol response compared with controls (Sinha, 2008). In these studies, this research group found that cocaine-dependent and alcohol-dependent individuals show increased anxiety and negative emotions during drug-cue exposure, while social drinkers report lower levels of negative affect and anxiety with alcohol-cue exposure. Thus, these studies show increased drug craving and altered hedonic response to both stress and drug cues in addicted individuals compared with social drinkers.

As addressed in Chapter 4, functional MRI studies have shown multiple brain regions associated with craving in addicted individuals. Exposure to drug cues known to increase craving increases activity in the amygdala, regions of the frontal cortex, hippocampus, insula, and VTA. Furthermore, stress-related stimuli, such as foot-shock, restraint stress, and anxiety-producing drugs, increase nucleus accumbens dopamine release (Imperato, 1992; McCullough, 1992; Kalivas, 1995); therefore, dopamine release in the nucleus accumbens likely mediates the conditioned reinforcement effects of both appetitive (to attract) and aversive (to avoid) stimuli in their ability to produce drug seeking behavior (Salamone, 1997).

Other evidence demonstrates the involvement of the amygdala in conditioned reinforcement effects of drugs associated stimuli. Amygdala nuclei are essential in the acquisition of Pavlovian fear conditioning (LeDoux, 2000), and stress exposure is known to increase dopamine release in the amygdala (Inglis, 1999). Furthermore, studies have shown that amygdala lesions disrupt conditioned drug seeking for cocaine and impair cue-mediated acquisition and reinstatement of drug seeking in rats (Whitelaw, 1996; Meil, 1997). Another research group (See, 2001) reported that the conditioned reinstatement of drug seeking is dependent on dopamine D1 receptors in the amygdala. Functional MRI brain imaging studies of drug abusers have shown that exposure to drug cues known to increase craving resulted in activation of the amygdala and regions of the frontal cortex (Grant, 1996; Childress, 1999; Kilts, 2001). Additional functional MRI brain imaging studies examining brain activation during stress and neutral imagery revealed increased medial temporal lobe (amygdala) and decreased frontal activation during stress imagery in cocaine-dependent individuals as compared with controls (Sinha, 2000b). These data suggest that the amygdala, which is anatomically linked to both the regions of the prefrontal cortex and the nucleus accumbens, plays a key role in conditioned emotional responding and affective learning (Gaffan, 1993; Dias, 1996; LeDoux, 2000) and is intimately involved in mediating the effects of stress and drug cues on drug craving.

Stress-Induced Reinstatement of Drug-Seeking Behavior and Relapse

Exposure to stress, drug-related stimuli, and drugs themselves reinstates drug-seeking behavior in animals and increases relapse susceptibility in addicted individuals (Sinha, 2007; Shaham, 2005; Weiss, 2005). Recently there have been a number of studies that have shown that brain CRF, noradrenergic (catecholamine), and glutaminergic pathways contribute to reinstatement of drug seeking and relapse (Marinelli, 2007; Mantsch, 2008, George, 2007). These studies have shown that neuroadaptations associated with chronic drug use result in overactive brain CRF and HPA axis responses, altered autonomic nervous system responses, altered glutaminergic pathways, and underactive dopamine and GABA pathways. These neuroadaptations lead to high craving states and relapse susceptibility. Consistent with this are animal studies that have used CRF, noradrenergic, and glutaminergic antagonists in reducing stress-induced seeking in addicted laboratory animals (Zhao, 2006; Aujla, 2007). All these studies are consistent with high distress and craving states associated with altered biological responses that regulate stress, craving, and impulse control.

Several animal studies have shown that stress reinstates drug-seeking behavior: Brief foot-shock or tail-pinch stress has been shown to increase drug-seeking behavior in abstinent, drug-addicted rats (Shaham, 1995; Erb, 1996; Ahmed, 1997; Le, 1998; Mantsch, 1999), and that stress-induced drug seeking can be blocked by CRF antagonists (Erb, 1998; Shaham, 1998). Furthermore, alpha 2-adrenergic agonists, which inhibit norepinephrine (NE) activity centrally, have been found to reduce stress-induced relapse to drug seeking (Erb, 2000; Shaham, 2000). These data show that brain CRF and NE circuits are directly involved in stress-induced drug seeking in addicted animals.

Human studies have shown that drug abusers and alcoholics often cite stress and negative affect as reasons for relapse to drug use (Marlatt, 1980, 1985; Bradley, 1989; Wallace 1989; McKay, 1995). Failure to cope with stress is associated with relapse in recovering alcoholics (Brown, 1990; Hodgkins, 1995); heroin addicts (Marlatt, 1980; Brewer, 1998), and recovering cocaine addicts (Sinha, 1999b). However, the mere occurrence of stressful life events is not, in itself, predictive of relapse (Hall, 1991; Miller, 1996).

Recently, Dr. Sinha's research group followed cocaine- and alcohol-dependent patients recently discharged from a residential treatment facility for ninety days to assess relapse outcomes. For abstinent cocaine addicts, they found that the magnitude of stress-induced cocaine craving in the laboratory significantly predicted time to cocaine relapse. While stress-induced ACTH and cortisol responses were not associated with time to relapse, these laboratory findings were predictive of amounts of cocaine consumed during follow-up (Sinha, 2006). In the same study group, drug cue–induced craving was not predictive of relapse. There was, however, a high correlation between stress and drug cue–induced drug craving, and stress and drug cue–induced HPA axis responses. These data suggest that at least in the case of cocaine dependence, stress and drug cue–induced stress produce similar relapse vulnerability.

In abstinent alcoholics, Sinha's group found that negative mood, stress-induced alcohol craving, blunted stress, and cue-induced cortisol responses significantly associated with alcohol relapse rates (Adinoff, 2005). Another research group from the University of Minnesota School of Medicine found that nicotine-deprived recovering smokers exposed to a series of stressors showed blunted ACTH, cortisol, and blood pressure responses to stress but high nicotine withdrawal and craving scores, and these responses were predictive of smoking relapse rates (Al'absi, 2005).

Thus, for recovering alcoholics and cocaine and smoking addicts, researchers conclude that the drug-craving state marked by increasing distress and craving along with poor stress regulatory responses (altered cortisol feedback or increased noradrenergic arousal) results in an enhanced susceptibility to addiction relapse. In addition, there is substantial evidence that stress, as well as addiction, impairs decision-making and judgment, further increasing relapse risk.

Stress-Induced Cognitive Impairment

Additional regions connected to the mesolimbic dopamine pathways involved in reward and learning (the amygdala, hippocampus, insula, and parts of the frontal lobe) play an important role in interoception (emotional interpretation) and stress processing, impulse control and decision-making. CRF, cortisol, and catecholamines target these pathways to induce adaptive and coping processes. For example, different parts of the medial prefrontal cortex are involved in higher cognitive or executive control functions, such as controlling and inhibiting impulses, regulating distress, focusing and shifting attention, monitoring behavior, linking behaviors and consequences over time, considering alternatives before acting, and making decisions. Psychosocial and behavioral scientists have repeatedly shown that with chronically elevated levels of emotional and physiological stress, there is a decrease in behavioral control and increases in impulsivity. Furthermore, with increasing severity and chronicity of stress, there is a greater risk of abnormal maladaptive behaviors and consequences (arrests, etc) (Barkley, 1997; Tice, 2001; Hayaki, 2005). In this regard, researchers have emphasized the importance of distinguishing the adaptive nature of acute stress fear conditioning from the maladaptive effects of severe and chronic stress on learning.

Neurobiological evidence has shown that with increasing levels of stress, there is a decrease in prefrontal functioning and increased limbic-level responding, which perpetuates low behavioral and cognitive control (Arnsten, 1998; Li, 2008). Given that both stress and drugs of abuse activate the mesolimbic pathways, it is not surprising that each results in synaptic adaptations in VTA dopamine neurons with *increased* quantity and quality of nerve connections, associated with reward center reinforcing neuroadaptations of addiction. Both chronic stress and drugs of abuse also cause morphological changes in the medial prefrontal cortex (PFC) with *decreased* quality and quantity of nerve connections, which are associated with learning disorders in these animals (Robinson, 1999; Liston, 2006) and observed in humans (more in Chapter 6). Similar adverse neuroadaptations are also seen in the hippocampus associated with chronic stress (Gurvits, 1996). High levels of cortisol receptors are found in the hippocampus and PFC. Consistent with these observations, studies have shown that early-life stress and prolonged and repeated stress early in life reduce cognitive performance later in life (Gratton, 2005). *Cortisol also adversely affect development of the PFC, a region that is highly dependent on environmental experiences for maturation The PFC, and particularly the right PFC, plays an important role both in activating the HPA axis and autonomic responses to stress and in regulating these responses (Gratton, 2005).* For example, lesions of the inferior frontal cortex, the orbitofrontal cortex, result in enhanced HPA axis and autonomic responses to stress. Thus, the decision-making and motivational brain pathways, as well as the reward centers are targets of brain stress chemicals and provide an important potential mechanism by which stress affects addiction vulnerability.

Psychologists have demonstrated that stress interferes with cognitive performance, particularly in the ability to sustain attention and in inhibition of goal-directed responses to stimuli (Glass, 1969, 1971; Hockey, 1970; Cohen, 1980). Some earlier research has shown that stress prevents the acquisition or execution of coping responses in affectively vulnerable individuals (Rosen, 1982; Faust, 1984). Lesions of the prefrontal cortex result in impaired sustained attention and response inhibition (Perret 1974; Wilkins, 1987). Stress and depression have been shown to increase impulsivity and decrease self-control (Muraven, 2000). Arnsten (1998) showed that noise stress impairs prefrontal cognitive function in monkeys, which is modulated by prefrontal dopaminergic pathways. Severe emotional stress is associated with loss of control over impulses and an inability to inhibit inappropriate behaviors and to delay gratification (Tice, 2001; Mischel, 1989; Muraven, 2000). Neurobiological data indicate that stress impairs catecholamine modulation of prefrontal circuits, which in turn impairs executive functions, like working memory and self-control (Arnsten, 1998a, 1998b, 2005).

There are a number of studies that have shown that adolescents at risk for substance abuse who have experienced cumulative psychosocial stressors are more likely to show decreased emotional and behavioral control, and that decreased self-control is associated with risk of substance abuse and other maladaptive behaviors (Wills, 2002, 2006, 2007; Baler, 2006). Adolescents at risk for substance abuse are known to have decreased executive functioning, low behavioral and emotional control, poor decision-making, and greater levels of deviant behavior and impulsivity (Fishbein, 2006; Baler, 2006; Giancola, 1996, 1998). Stress or drug alterations in the cortico-striatal-limbic dopamine pathways have been associated with impulsivity, decision-making, and addiction risk (Jentsch, 2003; Everitt, 2005). Specifically, the VTA, NA, PFC, and amygdala, are highly susceptible to stress-related signaling and plasticity associated with early-life stress and chronic stress experiences. In a recent PET imaging study, Oswald (2007) examined the effects of chronic stress and impulsivity on amphetamine-induced striatal dopamine release. The findings of this study indicated that impulsivity was associated with blunted VS dopamine and this effect was modified by a significant interaction with chronic psychosocial stress. With low to moderate stress, dopamine release was greater in low-impulsive than in high-impulsive subjects, but with high stress, both groups showed low dopamine release. These findings illustrate the important effects of stress on frontal lobe, striatal, and limbic dopamine transmission, and that psychosocial stress needs to be carefully considered to understand fully the role of stress on impulsivity and addiction risk.

Compromise of the hippocampus with stress also appears to be part of the loss of executive function and control in stress and drug addiction. As we discussed in Chapter 4, the hippocampus is the center of new memory formation. Cortisol works with epinephrine (adrenaline) to create memories of short-term emotional events; this is the proposed mechanism for storage of acute stress-related "flash-bulb" memories, and may originate as a means to remember what to avoid in the future. However, long-term exposure to cortisol impairs memory by damaging cells in the hippocampus. (Hippocampal atrophy was initially recognized in Cushing's syndrome, a primary adrenal disorder resulting in high levels of cortisol in the bloodstream.) The hippocampus contains high levels of cortisol receptors, which make it more vulnerable to long-term stress than most other brain areas. Stress-related steroids affect the hippocampus in at least three ways: first, by reducing the excitability of some hippocampal neurons; second, by inhibiting the genesis of new neurons; and third, by causing atrophy of neuronal connections (dendrites). There is evidence that humans who have experienced severe, long-lasting traumatic stress, show atrophy of the hippocampus, more than of other parts of the brain. These effects show up in post-traumatic stress disorder, and they may contribute to the hippocampal atrophy reported in schizophrenia, severe depression and chronic alcoholism. At least some of these effects appear to be reversible if the stress is discontinued.

Chapter 6

Cognitive Impairment from Addiction

William G.: I Can't Be That Stupid?

William G., about sixty years old, is a top-notch CEO of a large technology firm in Minnesota with over two hundred employees. He graduated top of his class from an Ivy League college and has a PhD from an elite California technology school. He is considered by many to be a genius. He has a loving family, lives in a large home, and owns several luxury cars. William is also an alcoholic who has been drinking daily for over thirty years. In the last fifteen years, he has drunk about a pint to a fifth of scotch (usually refined single malts) every day. He would drink heavily after a hard day at the office and would frequently sneak a shot (or two) in the morning and during work hours to steady his nerves. His work remained top-notch, but his family life was suffering under the weight of his alcoholism. He often made careless personal decisions and had memory lapses. His caring family finally intervened, and he entered a residential treatment center. Soon after admission he was administered a test of cognitive function, testing his memory and reasoning ability with mathematical and verbal problems. He scored in the bottom 20 percent of the country on that test. "I can't be that stupid," he claimed. After eight weeks of abstinence in the treatment program, he retook the test, scoring more than a full standard deviation higher, now in the top 33 percent of the country. Today, two years sober, he is a genius once more.

The Addict or Alcoholic Is the Last to Know

William's cognitive impairment is common, not only in alcoholics, but also at least in some degree in all individuals who are substance dependent.

Addicted individuals are often not aware of their own cognitive impairment because, well, they are impaired. They suffer real-life problems in memory, judgment, and decision-making. Many times these impairments are cleverly hidden from work associates and family members. This is not surprising, as mood-altering chemicals hijack the limbic reward centers of the brain, the origin of decision-making, emotions, and memory.

A hallmark of addiction is the compulsive use of a mind-altering substance despite negative consequences (i.e., poor decision-making). To a normal person, the decisions made by the alcoholic or addict frequently appear insane, as they pursue their addiction at the expense of family, reputation, financial security, and personal safety. Studies have consistently shown that individuals addicted to alcohol, cocaine, and methamphetamine, pursue actions that bring immediate reward at the risk of incurring future negative consequences (Bechara, 2002a, 2004; Scott, 2007; Verdejo-García, 2007a, 2007b). One study author described the actions of addicted individuals as "myopic for the future" (Rogers, 2001). The addict's actions are compulsive and uninhibited.

Numerous studies have shown that chronic drug abuse, as well as stress itself, has been shown to impair decision making, memory, and executive cognitive function. As addressed in the preceding chapters, the addict and alcoholic suffer from neuroadaptations and hormonal imbalances. Such neuroadaptations result in increased dopamine transmission in the reward centers and decreased dopamine release in the prefrontal cortex with addictive substances or with stress (Sorg, 1993, 1997; Kalivas, 1998; Prasad, 1999). The substance dependent individual also has hormonal imbalances due to a dysfunctional hypothalamic-pituitary-adrenal (HPA) axis. *This results in chronic elevation of the stress hormone, cortisol, that contributes to decreased functioning of the frontal lobes of the brain, which are necessary to carry out executive control functions.*

Other factors, which are somewhat drug specific, also contribute to cognitive decline in the addict and alcoholic. This chapter elaborates on the findings of multiple research studies and describes the neural pathways responsible for the decline in cognitive function and emotional appraisal in the addict and alcoholic.

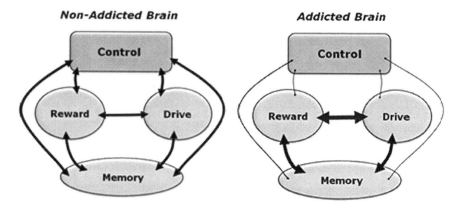

Non-Addicted Brain   **Addicted Brain**

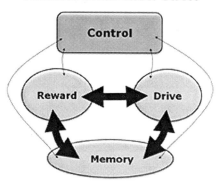

Addicted Brain Under Stress

The illustration above shows the progressive deterioration of control functions (decision-making, judgment, etc.) in addiction and acceleration of this deterioration with stress. In the non-addicted brain, there is balance between control centers and centers of reward and (motivation) drive. In the addicted brain, neuroadaptations and hormonal changes result in decreased control (inhibition) at the expense of increased drive for immediate reward (compulsion). With stress, either from external circumstances or from drug use or withdrawal itself, these changes are magnified, leading to further loss of control and inhibition. *Given the severe compromise of executive control functions, the vortex of addiction is viciously self-perpetuating and, therefore, life-threatening.*

Impaired Executive Functioning with Addiction

The addiction literature has shown repeatedly that addicts and alcoholics) have been shown to have deficits in the domain of *"executive functioning"* (Verdejo-García, 2006, 2007c). Executive functioning is a complex construct that involves different cognitive domains. Executive functioning involves the ability to make decisions; plan, judge, and weigh several options; have an accurate perception of one's own abilities; and organize, implement, and control other cognitive functions, such as memory and emotions (Oscar-Berman 2007; Tranel 1994, Verdejo-Garcia 2006).

The particular substance abused affects which particular aspect of executive function is impaired most severely (Selby, 1998). Gonzalez (2007b) directly compared performance of alcoholics and methamphetamine-addicted individuals on a decision-making test (Iowa Gambling Task) and test of working-memory task (delayed non-match to sample test). His group found that the effects of alcohol on these measures were milder than the effects of methamphetamine (see also Bechara, 2004; Verdejo-García, 2007a). On the same note, chronic alcohol abuse seems to have less of an effect on executive functioning than does cocaine abuse (Easton, 1997). Unless alcoholism is severe, the deficits in tests of memory, fluency, cognitive flexibility, and perseverative responding are generally relatively mild (Oscar-Berman, 2007). In contrast, chronic methamphetamine use, for example, has been associated with persistent and rather severe cognitive impairments in various domains of executive functioning (Barr, 2006). *These differences are likely due to the vascular constriction induced by the stimulants, leading to small strokes.*

Chronic users of benzodiazepines show significant impairments in working memory and less severe impairments in other cognitive functions (Lucki, 1986; Buffet-Jerrot 2002). Heavy marijuana users show impairments that are more general in executive functions, including attention, memory and decision-making (Pope, 1996). Opiate addicts show impairments in poor impulse control, planning, and decision-making (Prosser, 2006).

Impaired Decision Making in Addiction

Decision-making is a domain of executive functioning that is consistently impaired in individuals with a history of chronic drug or alcohol use. A number of studies that used similar decision-making paradigms have shown impairments in decision-making performance among alcohol, cannabis, cocaine, opiate, and methamphetamine abusers (Bechara, 2001; Grant, 2000; Heiman, 2002; Kirby, 1999; Monterosso, 2001; Paulus, 2002, 2003; Petry, 1998; Rogers, 1999). Several similar decision-making paradigms have been used in these studies, including tasks of delayed discounting (Kirby, 1999; Monterosso, 2001), betting tasks (Rogers, 1999), and probabilistic choice tasks (Paulus, 2002, 2003).

The most frequently used paradigm to assess decision-making is the Iowa Gambling Task (IGT), which was initially developed to investigate the decision-making defects of neurological patients (Bechara, 2001). The IGT requires the integration of different aspects of executive functioning in order for successful completion (Dunn, 2006). The key feature of the task is that participants have to forgo high short-term rewards (i.e., facsimile money) for long-term profit (Bechara, 2000). This task factors a number of aspects: immediate rewards and delayed punishments, risk, and uncertainty of outcomes (Bechara, 2003). Briefly, in the IGT, participants have to choose between decks of cards that yield high immediate gain but larger future loss, and decks that yield lower immediate gain but a smaller future loss (Bechara, 1994, 2002). It is important to note that in this task, it is difficult for an individual to keep track of the rewards and punishments encountered in each deck, and therefore, performance in the task is not entirely based on computations of the net value of each deck; i.e., it is difficult to "card count" the decks).

An active research group from the University of Southern California (Drs. Verdejo-Garcia, Bechara, Recknor, and Perz-Garcia, 2006b) proposed that participants respond to emotional signals obtained from prior experiences of reward and punishment. *These emotional signals are often unconscious to the individual in whom they are enacted, albeit are described as a "hunch" or a "gut feeling" that a given choice may be good or bad* (Bechara, 1997; Crone, 2004). These researchers refer to psycho-physiological (Bechara 2000, 2002b) and cognitive models (Stout, 2004, 2005) supporting their hypothesis that emotional factors associated with the processing of reward and punishment play a significant role in the decision-making performance on the IGT.

In a series of studies using the IGT, this research group compared the performance of active addicts with patients with damage to the orbitofrontal cortex (Bechara, 2002a, 2002b). These studies measured the participant's skin conductance response (as is used in lie-detector tests) as a physiological measure of autonomic activity. The physiological responses triggered after making the choice and seeing the outcome (i.e., gain or loss of facsimile money) were called "reward/punishment responses," and those generated before making the choice were called "anticipatory responses." These studies showed that good performance in the IGT was linked to the development of these anticipatory emotional responses, especially before selecting cards from the disadvantageous decks, suggesting that these anticipatory emotional responses help guide decision-making away from disadvantageous choices (Bechara, 1997, 2000; Crone, 2004).

In their 2002 study, Dr. Bechara's group distinguished between two types of individuals in their group of addicts (Bechara, 2002a). One type of addict (a minority of the sample) showed a behavioral profile similar to that of healthy participants (i.e., they selected more cards from the advantageous decks). They also showed a physiological profile similar to healthy participants, in that they began to trigger anticipatory SCRs *before* selecting cards from the bad decks. *By contrast, another type of addict (a majority of the sample) exhibited behavioral and physiological profiles that were different from healthy participants, and more similar to patients with orbitofrontal cortex damage. These addicts chose disadvantageously on the task, and they failed to acquire anticipatory skin conduction responses before choosing.*

In a later study, the research group used a variant version of the IGT (Bechara, 2002b): In this study, they reversed the order of reward and punishment contingencies, so that the advantageous decks yielded high immediate punishment and even higher future reward, and the disadvantageous decks had lower immediate punishment, and even lower long-term reward. Using this IGT protocol, they found addicts who were hypersensitive to immediate reward and those who were insensitive to long-term consequences.

Thus, in Bechara's series of studies they found three groups of addicts: first, a small subpopulation of addicts who were behaviorally and physiologically indistinguishable from healthy participants; second, a small subpopulation that was indistinguishable from orbitofrontal lesion patients; and third, a larger sub-population of addicts, who were different from the other two and exhibited signs of hypersensitivity to reward and insensitivity to long-term consequences. These three groups did not differ in terms of basic original cognitive abilities, severity, or duration of drug use.

Other research groups have replicated this pattern of behavioral and physiological response using the Cambridge Gamble Task paradigm, which isolates different components of the IGT (Clark, 2002; Fishbein, 2005). In Fishbein's 2005 study, polydrug users selected more risky choices in the high-risk conditions of the task, and failed to generate increased skin conduction responses when making riskier decisions with regard to healthy participants. Different studies using the IGT have shown that poorer decision-making performance in addicts is associated with abnormal generation of anticipatory emotional responses, which precede the selection of cards from high-risk decks.

Notable to this discussion, is that abnormal triggering and possible procession of markers of autonomic function (emotional signals) also have been reported in healthy, non-addicted participants who perform poorly in the IGT (Crone, 2004; Suzuki, 2008). *Dr. Verdejo-Garcia went on to hypothesize that at least some of the decision-making alterations observed in addicts may have actually preceded the drug abuse stage and are a predisposing factor that contributed to the switch from casual drug use to a compulsive and uncontrolled addiction problem.*

This hypothesis becomes pertinent in view of the fact that even among drug naive individuals, there are individual differences in the capacity to make advantageous decisions, including sensitivity to reward/insensitivity to punishment, and in decision-making performance as measured by the IGT (Crone, 2004; Suzuki, 2008). This raises the question of whether these "emotional" and decision-making measures serve as markers of future addiction. Decision-making deficits have also been reported in populations who are at high risk for drug abuse, such as adolescents with externalizing behavior disorders (Ernst, 2002), and individuals with Antisocial Personality Disorder (APD) (Mazas, 2000; Mitchell, 2002), a psychiatric disorder that is robustly associated with substance dependence and which involves severe disturbances in emotion processing. Impaired decision-making is also observed in individuals under chronic stress and those with chronically elevated cortisol levels (Chapter 5).

Overall, these studies support the hypothesis that impaired decision-making in addiction is associated with altered reactions to rewarding and punishing events, as well as altered elicitation and processing of emotional signals that help forecast or anticipate the consequences of future events. Although all researchers agree that impaired decision making follows substance abuse, some hypothesize it may actually precede it and make an individual at risk for substance abuse.

Impaired Emotion Processing in Addiction

There are a substantial number of studies that have examined impaired emotional perception (interoception) and its relationship to impaired decision-making in addicted individuals. Most studies on emotional perception and appraisal have focused on the manner in which addicts and alcoholics interpret emotional facial expressions (Hoshi, 2004; Kano, 2002; Kornreich, 2001, 2003). A study by Dr. Kornreich (2001) of Brugman Hospital in Belgium showed that alcohol dependent individuals showed specific impairments for recognizing facial expressions portraying happiness and anger. The alcoholics tended to overestimate the intensity of the emotion depicted in these emotional facial expressions. These findings have been replicated in abstinent alcoholics and opiate addicts, and in opiate addicts undergoing methadone treatment (Konreich, 2003). Dr. Townshend of the University of Sussex, England, showed that overestimation of the intensity of emotion in facial expressions reported by alcoholics related mainly to the facial expression of fear. In his study, alcoholics also presented with difficulties in distinguishing between the facial expressions of anger and disgust (Townshend, 2003). Interestingly, the degree of overestimation correlated with the number of previous formal detoxifications.

Other studies have analyzed the effects of acute usage of different drugs on the perception of emotions (Hoshi, 2004; Kano, 2002). These studies have shown that acute low doses of alcohol and the designer drug, MDMA, can improve the recognition of emotional facial expressions in active users, although recognition accuracy significantly decreased during the following abstinent days. Detrimental effects of acute drug doses on the recognition of emotions in facial expressions have also been reported using the dissociative drug, ketamine, an NMDA receptor (for glutamate) antagonist (Abel, 2003).

The authors of these studies hypothesize that addicts and alcoholics are impaired in the recognition of facial expressions portraying different emotions, including fear, anger, disgust, and happiness and that this limits their interpretation of social cues. The addict and alcoholic, therefore, are less able to make decisions and solve problems of an interpersonal or social nature, and this impairment further limits their ability to manage and regulate emotions.

In this regard, their poor ability to recognize facial emotional expressions explains other behaviors of the addict and alcoholic, such as diminished empathy and increased levels of aggression (Hoshi, 2004; Townshend, 2003). In particular, the poor recognition of fear expressions can be associated with a more generalized impaired conditioned of fear responses, a function of the amygdala. This generalized abnormal fear response can be extended to lack of fear of the consequences of drug use or drug-related environments, increasing the likelihood of relapses.

Researchers have also studied the emotional experience of the addict using the presentation of affective images that induce emotional states, such as those in the International Affective Picture System (IAPS) (Gerra, 2003). The IAPS consists of a large set of images classified according to their normative values in three relevant dimensions: valence (indicating if the emotional response induced is pleasant or unpleasant), arousal (if the emotional response induced is arousing or relaxing), and control (if the emotional response induced can/cannot be controlled by the subject). Dr. Gerra (2003) used this paradigm to analyze the neuroendocrine response of substance dependent individuals and healthy participants to experimentally induced pleasant and unpleasant emotions. *Their results showed that in response to unpleasant images, active addicts showed decreased activity in several neuroendocrine markers, including norepinephrine, cortisol, and adrenocorticotropic hormone levels.* Other research groups have replicated Dr. Gerra's findings (Aguilar, 2004). In these studies, addicts and alcoholics showed a more flattened response pattern to both pleasant and unpleasant images. Addicts and alcoholics scored as less positive the images considered by normal participants to be very pleasant and arousing and less negative the images considered by normal participants to be highly unpleasant and arousing.

Researchers hypothesize that the fact that addicts and alcoholics showed a flattened emotional response to affective images showing both pleasant and aversive scenes may suggest that they also have a diminished emotional response to natural stimuli, other than drugs, because drugs and alcohol possess exaggerated rewarding effects. This notion is strongly supported by imaging studies on craving in drug addiction, which show that drug-related stimuli are able to activate strongly brain regions involved in emotional evaluation and reward processing (Garavan, 2000; George, 2001; Kilts, 2002, 2004; Wang, 1999; Wexler, 2001). In contrast, the same brain regions show blunted activation to other natural reinforcing stimuli, such as food or sex (Garavan, 2000). Consistent with this evidence, other authors propose that emotional states associated with natural rewards may not be strong enough to bias decisions in addicts and alcoholics, while strong emotional states are associated with the prospect of abusing drugs or alcohol (Verdejo-Garcia, 2006).

Impaired Working Memory with Substance Dependence

Research investigating the effects of alcohol and drugs of abuse on memory is vast in animal and human populations. *The available evidence clearly indicates that ethanol and abused drugs significantly affect memory processes.* Studies of addicts and alcoholics have suggested that deficits in the working-memory domain are not purely due to a mnemonic impairment. Rather, impairments may be due to an executive control problem, namely decision-making and response inhibition. Specifically, Bechara and Martin (2004) found that individuals addicted to alcohol, cocaine, or methamphetamine performed below normal levels on the working-memory task, but increasing the memory load did not influence performance. The task used in this study (i.e., the delayed non-match to sample; DNMS) includes a memory component and an executive component. Because performance of addicts and alcoholics was not influenced by increased memory load, the authors argued that the deficiency in addicts and alcoholics displayed on this task must be related to the executive component of working memory as opposed to the storage component. Thus, according to these and other authors, problems in addicts and alcoholics arise when a strategy should be efficiently implemented to memorize items (Bechara and Martin, 2004; Woods, 2005; Scott, 2007). Van der Plas (2009) found that cocaine—and methamphetamine-dependent individuals were impaired on complex decision-making, working memory, and cognitive flexibility, but not on response inhibition. The deficits in working memory and cognitive flexibility were milder than the decision-making deficits and did not change as a function of memory load or task switching.

Memory Impairments with Specific Drug Types

Multiple studies in animals and humans have shown that alcohol primarily disrupts the ability to form new long-term memories. Alcohol causes less disruption of recall of previously established long-term memories than the ability to keep new information active in short-term memory for a few seconds or more (Acheson, 1998; Bliss, 1993; Eichenbaum, 2002; Givens, 1997; Goodwin, 1969a, 1970, 1995). At low doses, the impairments produced by alcohol are often subtle, though they are detectable in controlled conditions, such as test taking. As the amount of alcohol consumed increases, so does the magnitude of the memory impairments. Large quantities of alcohol, particularly if consumed rapidly, can produce a blackout, an interval of time for which the intoxicated person cannot recall key details of events or even entire events (Mello, 1973).

Tremendous progress has been made toward an understanding of the mechanisms underlying alcohol-induced memory impairments. *Alcohol has been found to disrupt activity in the hippocampus via several routes.* Alcohol affects the hippocampus directly, leading to atrophy after chronic ingestion (Agarst, 1999), and indirectly, by interfering with interactions between the hippocampus and other brain regions (Bliss, 1993; Blitzer, 1990; Silvers, 2003). The impact of alcohol on the frontal lobes remains poorly understood, but probably plays an important role in alcohol-induced memory impairments.

Alcohol-induced amnesia is mediated by stimulating the GABA transmitter system and activating the benzodiazepine/GABA receptor complex (Morrisett, 1993; Schummer, 2001). The GABA system is inhibitory and accounts for the sedative effects of alcohol. This is consistent with extensive evidence that benzodiazepines also induce amnesia in humans and laboratory animals. Chronic administration of high doses of alcohol to rats or mice over time induces memory impairment, accompanied by a decreased function of cholinergic systems in specific brain regions, including the hippocampus and neocortex. Such findings suggest that the memory impairment resulting from chronic ethanol ingestion is also associated with a deficit of brain cholinergic function (Adermark, 2001; Nardone, 2010).

Clinical research shows that chronic ingestion of alcohol can produce three general categories of severe cognitive impairment that are associated with memory deficits: the Wernicke-Korsakoff syndrome, alcoholic dementia, and "nonamnesiac" or "non-Korsakoff" disorders (Goodwin, 1995). Wernicke-Korsakoff syndrome, the best known, is due to vitamin B$_1$ (thiamine) deficiency, resulting from poor food intake during sustained periods of alcohol consumption. Most people who recover from an acute phase after treatment with thiamine will have residual Korsakoff's syndrome, in which there is an impairment of the ability to learn and remember new information (antegrade amnesia), as well as retention of recently acquired information (retrograde amnesia). Interestingly, these individuals apparently maintain near-normal intellectual function and the ability to acquire and retain skill-based information, such as purely visual/ motor tasks, like driving a car. Some improvement in the memory deficits may occur with prolonged abstinence from alcohol.

Alcoholic dementia differs from Korsakoff's syndrome in that it is characterized by severe memory impairment as well as major intellectual deterioration that can be difficult to distinguish from Alzheimer's disease. Improvements are, however, often seen if patients abstain from alcohol. The changes seen in late alcoholic dementia, like those of Alzheimer's disease, involve multiple brain regions, primarily in the temporal and frontal lobes, but also in other brain regions, and involve deficits in glutaminergic, GABAergic, and cholinergic systems (Kopelman, 2009).

The third type of memory problem linked to alcohol ingestion has been variously referred to as "neurologically intact" or "neurologically asymptomatic" and is characterized by subtle impairments in dealing with abstractions, problem solving, and memory. This form of memory problem is typical in moderate to heavy social drinkers and "functional" alcoholics. Significant recovery with abstinence is typical.

Benzodiazepines adversely affect multiple areas of cognition, the most notable one being that it interferes with the formation and consolidation of new memories and may induce complete antegrade amnesia (Ballenger, 2000). Like alcohol, benzodiazepines stimulate the GABA neurotransmitter system on the benzodiazepine/GABA receptor complex. Their effects on memory appear to be mediated primarily by their effect on the hippocampus and related circuitry. Researchers hold contrary opinions regarding the effects of long-term administration. One view is that many of the short-term effects continue into the long-term and are not resolved after quitting benzodiazepines (Verdoux, 2005; Barker, 2004; Stewart, 2005). Another view maintains that cognitive deficits in chronic benzodiazepine users occur only for a short period after the dose, or that underlying anxiety disorders cause memory deficits. While the definitive studies are lacking, the former view has the best support in the addiction community.

Studies on cannabis and memory are hindered by small sample sizes, confounding drug use, and other factors. The strongest evidence regarding cannabis and memory focuses on its short-term negative effects on short-term and working memory (Riedel, 2005). In laboratory animals, both acute and chronic administration of marijuana extracts or of their active principles, tetrahydrocannabinol (THC), have been reported to impair the acquisition and retention of a very wide variety of tasks (Ranganathan, 2006). *In humans, researchers and clinicians agree that cannabinoids impair all aspects of short-term memory, especially short-term episodic and working memory* (Ranganathan, 2006). One small study found that no learning occurred during the two-hour period in which the subjects (infrequent users) were "stoned" (Curran, 2002). Cessation of marijuana use typically results in rapid recovery from the drug effects. Little is known about brain influences mediating marijuana effects on learning and memory.

Several studies have shown that opiates, specifically heroine and morphine, impair memory retention during training in laboratory animals (Kapp, 1979, Bruins-Slot, 1999; Lundqvist, 2010). In addition, the administration of opiates prior to training does not decrease the impairment. Opiate-receptor antagonists, including naloxone and naltrexone, enhance memory and block the memory impairment produced by opiates. Endogenous opiates (endorphins) also affect memory. Despite the widespread and long-standing use of opiate drugs by humans, there have been few systematic studies on the effect of morphine, heroin, or other opiates on human memory. *Available studies have shown that chronic opiate users show moderate memory deficits* (Ersche, 2006, 2007). Acute administration of opiates (as in pre-anesthetic medication, for example) may induce a temporary amnesia. Surgery patients frequently fail to remember experiences immediately prior to surgery. The effect of opiate antagonists has been explored clinically in the treatment of dementias, but with limited success.

In laboratory animals and humans, chronic administration of amphetamines, including the popular methamphetamine, leads to memory deficits (Meneses, 2011; Siegel, 2010; Marshall, 2007; Hruba, 2010). Such deficits are typically obtained in experiments using high doses of amphetamine and complex learning tasks. In contrast, several animal studies have shown that acute post-training injections of low-dose amphetamine produce dose-dependent enhancement of memory. Retention is also enhanced by direct administration of amphetamine into several brain regions, including the amygdala and hippocampus.

Human amphetamine users also report that memory is enhanced by acute doses and impaired by chronic use. Amphetamine is known to act by releasing the catecholamines epinephrine, norepinephrine, and dopamine from cells and block their reuptake. Amphetamine effects on memory appear to result primarily from influences on brain dopaminergic systems as well as influences on the release of peripheral catecholamines (Simon, 2010). Deterioration of memory function with chronic amphetamine use usually subsides with cessation of use (King, 2010; Simon, 2010). *The memory impairment seen with high-dose amphetamines also may be attributed to multiple small strokes throughout the brain, as amphetamines are powerful vasoconstrictors.*

Despite the extensive use and abuse of cocaine, little is known about cocaine effects on memory. Results of studies using rats and mice indicate that acute post-training administration induces dose-dependent effects comparable to those of amphetamine. Memory is enhanced by low doses and impaired by higher doses (Sudai, 2011). The brain processes mediating cocaine influences on memory have not been extensively investigated. The effects appear to be mediated by influences on adrenergic and dopaminergic systems. Also, as with amphetamine, users of cocaine report that memory is enhanced by acute doses and impaired by chronic use. Several research groups have demonstrated that elevated cortisol levels are associated with learning and memory deficits in cocaine-dependent individuals, and these cognitive deficits, in addition to other cocaine-related neuroadaptations, increases relapse rates after periods of abstinence (Fox, 2009, Moeller, 2010).

Neurobiology of Impaired Executive Function in Addiction

Neuropsychological and neuroimaging studies in humans, as well as lesion and electrophysiological studies in animals, suggest that executive functioning relies in large part on the prefrontal cortex (PFC) and its interactions with other brain regions (Stuss, 1986). These studies, together with studies reporting PFC neuronal loss in substance-dependent individuals (Adams, 1993; Krill, 1997), suggest that cognitive deficits observed in addicts and alcoholics may be associated with dysfunction of the PFC.

The PFC is heterogeneous in its functions and incorporates diverse abilities related to cognitive control functions such as working memory, cognitive flexibility, and response inhibition. Researchers have identified that functions of the PFC are integral to the formulation and execution of goal-directed actions (Stuss, 2002; Roberts, 1998) and the regulation of emotions (Bechara, 2000; Davidson, 2002). Three different functional circuits relevant to executive control and emotional regulation have been described: the dorsolateral prefrontal cortex (DLPFC), orbitofrontal cortex (OFC), and anterior cingulate cortex (ACC) circuits (Cummings, 1993; Tekin, 2002). Dysfunction within each PFC circuit is associated with different deficits.

Primary Brain Regions Involved in Cognitive Impairment

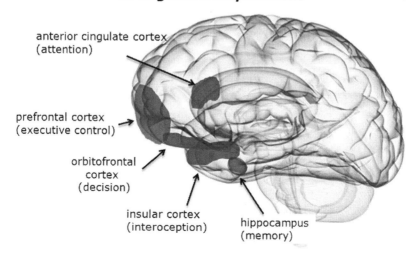

anterior cingulate cortex
(attention)

prefrontal cortex
(executive control)

orbitofrontal
cortex
(decision)

insular cortex
(interoception)

hippocampus
(memory)

The dorsolateral prefrontal cortex (DLPFC) is mainly associated with executive control, and patients with DLPFC lesions usually perform poorly on tests of working memory and mental flexibility (Bechara, 2000). For example, poorer performance on tests of working memory and cognitive flexibility, linked to the functioning of the DLPFC, has been reported in users of alcohol (Errico, 2002) and polysubstance users of amphetamines (Ornstein et al., 2000) and cocaine (Klüber, 2005). The DLPFC is thought to subserve working memory (Goldman-Rakic, 1992) and appears particularly important for the executive processor of mnemonic operations (Petrides, 2000). Brain imaging studies have shown increased activation of the DLPFC with drug craving (Grant, 1996; Bonson, 2002).

The anterior cingulate cortex (ACC) is associated with attention, motivation and initiative. Individuals with ACC lesions demonstrate defective performance on tests of response inhibition, including Go/No-Go tasks (Garavan, 2002; Tekin, 2002). Similarly, deficits in inhibitory control, linked to the functioning of the ACC, have been detected in users of alcohol (Fillmore, 2004) and polysubstance users of cocaine (Fillmore, 2002) and methamphetamine (Monterosso, 2005). The ACC is also activated in brain imaging studies of craving (Chapter 4).

An important region involved in processing many types of rewards and punishments and making rapid changes in response to environmental change is the orbitofrontal cortex (OFC). The OFC is associated with emotional regulation, stimulus reinforcement learning, and decision-making. Patients with damage to the OFC usually perform poorly on tests that involve emotional processing, reversal learning and decision-making (Bechara, 2000; Clark, 2004; Rolls, 2004). Deficits in emotional processing were also reported in addicts and alcoholics, including inaccurate perception of facial expressions (Hoshi, 2004; Townshend, 2003) and abnormal responses to affective images (Aguilar de Arcos, 2005; Gerra, 2003).

Several studies have shown OFC dysfunction in substance-dependent individuals (Adinoff, 2006; Breiter, 2001; Knutson, 2000; Tanabe, 2007). For example, using single photon emission computed tomography (SPECT), an imaging study that measures blood flow. Adinoff and colleagues (2006) showed that individuals addicted to cocaine had reduced activity in the OFC relative to healthy comparisons when performing the Iowa Gambling Task (IGT). The functional integrity of the OFC relies on neural systems that subserve memory, in particular working memory, which integrates the neural circuits of the hippocampus and insular cortex of the temporal lobe (Bechara and Tranel, 2002). Working memory is defined as the process of storing and online manipulation of information (Baddeley, 1994) and includes short-term storage, rehearsal and the executive processes that operate on the contents of memory (Smith, 1999).

Studies using neuroimaging techniques have demonstrated that substance dependence is associated with abnormalities in different key components of a PFC–striatal neural circuit (Franklin, 2002; Lim, 2002; Matochik, 2003). (Recall that the striatum includes the nucleus accumbens, the primary reward center.) Furthermore, several functional imaging studies have shown abnormal activation of PFC systems in response to cognitive and emotional tasks in users of multiple drugs (Bolla, 2003, 2004; Ersche, 2005; Fishbein, 2005; Garavan, 2000). Addicts and alcoholics present with behavioral problems that are similar to those observed in patients with damage to different functional components of the PFC. These problems include apathy, lack of initiative, and low motivation for natural reinforcers (linked to ACC; Kalechstein, 2002); poor emotional regulation, poor judgment, and impulsivity (linked to OFC; Bechara, 2001); and goal-neglect, disorganized behavior (linked to DLPC; Verdejo-García, 2004).

Functional MRI studies have shown that drug-dependent individuals show hypoactive brain responses to problem-solving errors (i.e., detecting when one makes a mistake) in both the ACC and the insular cortex of the temporal lobe (Forman, 2004; Kaufman, 2003). *Recall, the insular cortex is implicated in interoception, the perception of emotions.* Deficits in this rudimentary cognitive function may contribute to the cognitive deficits in users on risk-taking and learning tasks (Garavan, 2005). Indeed, stimulant users are less likely to make strategic shifts in performance (e.g., win-stay, lose-shift) and this is related to activation differences in the dorsolateral prefrontal cortex and the insula (Paulus, 2003, 2008).

It is notable that cocaine addicts and heavy cannabis users have been shown to have a poorer subjective awareness of performance errors (i.e., detecting when one makes a mistake) on a task designed specifically to assess error awareness (the Go/No-Go task) (Hester, 2009, 2010). This task requires subjects to indicate, by pressing a button, when they make an error-of-commission on a Go/No-Go task which contains two rules that dictate when to inhibit responding. The awareness of errors is distinct from overall performance on the task, suggesting a deficit that is separate from the poor inhibitory control already associated with drug use (Verdejo-Garcia, 2007). Neuroimaging data, currently only available on the cannabis users, links this awareness deficit to the functioning of the ACC and the insula (Hester, 2009). These deficits in subjective awareness of behavior are notable given (1) the evidence of volumetric deficiencies in the insula in drug users and (2) evidence that greater anterior insular volumes are linked to better subjective awareness of inner bodily states (Critchley, 2004). These cognitive deficits in monitoring and being consciously aware of one's behavior may have direct relevance to drug cravings. Compromised monitoring may result in drug users being poor to realize when they are exposing themselves to exogenous and endogenous craving triggers. For example, deficient monitoring might lead the user to high-risk situations containing drug availability or drug cues that might initiate craving.

Impaired Neural Circuits Processing Emotions in Addiction

The neural circuitry that is critical for decision-making overlaps considerably with that for processing emotions, as measured in complex laboratory decision-making tasks, such as the Iowa Gambling Test (IGT). In a PET activation study performed by Dr. Ernst of the NIH, which examined patterns of brain activation during IGT performance in healthy participants, the researchers observed that decision-making was associated with increased activation in the orbitofrontal, anterior cingulate, and parietal/insular cortices and the amygdala (Ernst, 2002). Other regions that were also activated during the performance of decision-making tasks included the dorsolateral prefrontal cortex, thalamus, and cerebellum. Later imaging studies have confirmed and extended these findings, and implicated additional neural regions (e.g., the striatum) (Verney, 2003) and the nucleus accumbens (Mathews, 2004) in processes that are critical for decision-making.

Dr. Bolla (2003), of the Johns Hopkins School of Medicine, used oxygen labeled PET to examine brain activation in twenty-five day abstinent cocaine-dependent patients while performing the IGT. Group analyses showed increased activation during gambling task performance in the right

OFC, and less activation in the left DLPFC cortex of cocaine patients, with regard to healthy subjects. Activation of the OFC was directly correlated with better performance of both groups, and negatively correlated with amount of cocaine used in the patient group. The authors suggested that the activation is representative of the "mental effort" applied to the task. In another study, Ersche (2005) tested current opiate and amphetamine users and ex-users in the Cambridge Gambling Task (Clarke, 2002), which was designed to isolate the evaluation of risky decision-making from the planning and working memory components inherent in the IGT. In this study, addicts and matched healthy comparison participants were imaged with oxygen-labeled PET while performing this decision-making task. Results revealed that drug abusers performing the risk task showed increased activation of the left OFC and decreased activation of the right DLPFC (identical localization but reversed lateralization with respect to the results of the Bolla 2003 study).

Other studies have employed functional MRI to examine patterns of brain regional activation in abstinent methamphetamine abusers using a two-choice prediction task (Paulus, 2003, 2008). In brief, this task labors the participant's decision-making function by requiring the prediction of an uncertain outcome. Unlike IGT, this task does not involve incentive evaluation of rewards and punishments. Imaging patterns in methamphetamine individuals while performing the two-choice prediction task showed decreased activation of the OFC, DLPFC, and insular and inferior parietal cortices. The deactivations were irrespective of success or failure at the task. Orbitofrontal activation was inversely correlated with duration of methamphetamine use (Paulus, 2003).

Dr. Franklin (2002), of the University of Pennsylvania School of Medicine performed MRI morphology analysis of structural changes on brain scans of cocaine-dependent individuals. This group found significant decrements in grey matter concentrations (ranging from 5 to 11 percent) in the OFC, ACC, insula, and superior temporal cortices. The reductions in grey matter volume were not significantly correlated with measures of severity of drug dependence. Matochik et al. (2003) used digital volume analyses to measure grey and white matter composition of the brains of abstinent cocaine-dependent individuals. However, these authors focused on the analysis of tissue composition in the frontal lobe and its main structural subdivisions: dorsolateral, cingulate, and orbitofrontal regions. Their results showed significant grey matter decrements in the lateral prefrontal cortex, cingulate cortex, and medial and lateral aspects of the orbitofrontal cortex, predominantly in the right hemisphere. This study also failed to report significant correlations between indices of severity of drug abuse and reductions in grey matter volume, although the years of cocaine use were associated with lower tissue density in the inferior white matter adjacent to the frontal cortex.

In a later study, Makris et al. (2004) specifically measured the volume of the amygdala on both sides using segmentation-based morphometric analysis in cocaine dependent individuals. They found decreased absolute volume, primarily in the right amygdala (23 percent volume reductions, although total volume was also decreased), covering nuclei of the centromedial and basolateral areas and absence of lateral asymmetry in the cocaine group. The reduced volumetric measures of the amygdala did not correlate with measures of drug use severity.

Other studies have focused on white matter microstructure (Lim, 2002; Bartzokis, 2005). White matter tracts are composed mainly of nerve axons (wires) and not nerve bodies. Bartzokis et al. (2005), in an MRI study comparing male cocaine-dependent individuals with healthy participants, showed a higher incidence of age-related white matter lesions within the insular cortex of the cocaine addicts. Using diffusion tensor MRI, which is highly sensitive to white matter lesions, Lim (2002) showed altered white matter microstructure in the inferior frontal regions. These abnormalities seem to reflect disruption of functional connectivity between the OFC and a number of perilimbic regions involved in the processing of emotional states, such as the insular cortex.

Other researchers found similar white matter abnormalities in prefrontal and insular regions in cocaine dependent individuals (Lyoo, 2004). A research group from the University of Texas used diffusion tensor MR imaging to show that cocaine-dependent individuals present with white matter abnormalities in the anterior region of the corpus callosum (large white matter tract connecting the right and left hemispheres of the brain), and that the severity of these abnormalities correlate with measures of impulsivity (Moeller, 2005). The authors suggest that the callosum abnormalities likely underlie frontal lobe dysfunction.

Using functional MRI, a group led by Dr. Chang (2002), from the Brookhaven National Laboratory, analyzed the regional cerebral blood flow of long-term abstinent methamphetamine-dependent individuals. Their results showed decreased regional CBF in the insular cortices and inferior frontal regions, bilaterally, and in the right lateral parietal region. In a study of ninety-four Ecstasy abusers, using PET-glucose imaging, researchers found functional abnormalities in the ACC, amygdala, striatum, and hippocampus (Obrocki, 2002). SPECT blood-flow studies consistently show multiple perfusion defects in cocaine abusers (Holman, 1992; Kosten, 2008).

Brain SPECT Blood-Flow Scans

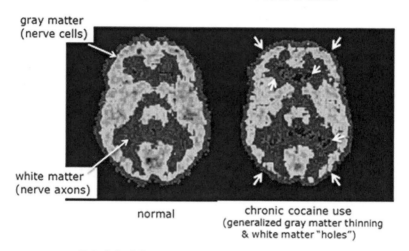

gray matter
(nerve cells)

white matter
(nerve axons)

normal

chronic cocaine use
(generalized gray matter thinning
& white matter "holes")

(Modified from Kosten, 2008, with permission)

Overall, the findings from both structural and functional imaging studies consistently indicate that several key neural substrates involved in executive function and emotional regulation are altered in addicted individuals. The inability of the addict or alcoholic to make proper decisions and manage emotions undermines his or her efforts to maintain sobriety.

Is Cognitive Impairment Reversible?

Studies measuring cognitive function after achieving abstinence are relatively sparse and varied and there are few long-term follow-ups. Longitudinal studies in this particular patient population are difficult. The best studies have been following alcoholics who have completed inpatient treatment. These studies have shown that certain alcohol-related cognitive impairment is reversible with abstinence (Volkow, 1995). Newly detoxified adult alcoholics often exhibit mild yet significant deficits in some cognitive abilities, especially problem-solving, short-term memory, and visuospatial abilities (Sullivan, 2000a). *By remaining abstinent, however, the recovering alcoholic will continue to recover brain function over a period of several months to one year (Sullivan, 200b), showing improvements in working memory, visuospatial functioning, and attention.* These changes are accompanied by significant increases in brain volume, compared with treated alcoholics who have subsequently relapsed to drinking (Sullivan, 2000a).

Brain imaging studies also show observable regression of alcohol and other drug-related injuries. Upon abstinence, partial reversal of brain volume loss associated with chronic alcoholism has been reported with CT and MRI (Carlen, 1978; Lishman, 1981) (Schroth, 1988; Zipursky, 1989; Bendszus, 2001). This brain volume regain upon abstinence indicates that cerebral tissue shrinking is not entirely due to irreversible neuronal damage. Although there is some evidence that morphological restitution can partially be attributed to rehydration (Mander, 1989; Trabert, 1995; Schroth, 1988), the overall brain volume gain attained early upon abstinence, its localization, and association with metabolic indicators for neuron growth from alcoholic brain damage indicate regeneration of nerves; their projections and measures of nerve regeneration correlate with improvements in measures of neuropsychological function (Mason, 2006; Gazdzinski, 2005a). Upon longitudinal studies with sobriety, evidence for recovering metabolites associated with nerve growth has been reported (Bendszu,s 2001; Parks, 2002; Durazzo, 2006; Bendszus, 2001; Ende, 2005). Interestingly, concomitant smoking and nicotine abuse are strongly suspected to exacerbate brain nerve cell loss in alcoholics (Durazzo, 2004) and to constrain their recovery upon abstinence (Durazzo, 2006).

Brain perfusion (blood flow in very small vessels) is abnormal in chronic cocaine and other stimulant users and is the primary reason for brain injury in this group. Basically, they get numerous small strokes. To determine whether these perfusion abnormalities are reversible following treatment, Holman (1992) studied cocaine-dependent polydrug users with SPECT blood flow imaging two to three days after admission to an inpatient treatment facility and at seven to eight days and seventeen to twenty-nine days after abstinence from drugs. This research group found a 5 to 20 percent improvement in blood flow in the addicts' first thirty days of treatment, showing that the perfusion defects observed in chronic cocaine polydrug users are partially reversible with short-term abstinence.

Neurogenesis and Neuroplasticity

Neurogenesis (birth of neurons) is the process by which neurons are formed, usually most robust in the womb (pre-natal development), although in recent decades has been identified in adult mammals and humans. Neurogenesis is responsible for populating the growing brain with neurons. *Neuroplasticity*, a term indicating that brain is "plastic" and "malleable," refers to the ability of the human brain to change because of one's experience. The discovery of this feature of the brain is rather modern. Neuroplasticity occurs through change in the strength of the connections, by adding or removing connections, and by the formation of new cells. Neuroplasticity is seen during repair from injury (physical or metabolic—i.e. substances of abuse) and with learning. Interestingly, injury and other pathology has been shown to not only stimulate adult neurogenesis in neurogenic regions, but also promote nerve cell growth in non-neurogenic regions (Arlotta et al., 2003; Parent, 2003).

Neurogenesis was traditionally believed to occur only during embryonic stages in the mammalian central nervous system (CNS) (Ramon and Cajal, 1913). *Only recently has it become generally accepted that new neurons are indeed added in discrete regions of the adult mammalian CNS* (Gross, 2000; Gould, 1999b; Kempermann,1999; Lie, 2004).

In most mammals, active neurogenesis occurs throughout life in the subventricular zone (SVZ) of the lateral ventricle (front and back corners of the water containing ventricles in the center of the brain) and in the subgranular zone (SGZ) of the hippocampus (center of new memories). Neurogenesis outside these two regions appears to be extremely limited in the intact adult mammalian CNS. After pathological stimulation, such as brain insults, adult neurogenesis appears to occur in regions otherwise considered non-neurogenic. New nerve cells are born in these areas and migrate to new areas injured or stimulated and then integrate (form synaptic connections) with existing cells and themselves (Alvarez-Buylla, 2004; Goh, 2003, Kempermann, 1999; Lie, 2004). The demonstration of active neurogenesis in adult humans not only shows the unforeseen regenerative capacity of the mature CNS, but also raises hopes for repairing the damaged adult CNS after injury or degenerative neurological diseases (Ming, 2005).

Electrical activity in stimulated neurons promotes neurogenesis. For example, excitatory nerve stimuli can be sensed by proliferating nerve cells via calcium channels and NMDA (glutamate) receptors (Deisseroth, 2004). Electrical activity also stimulates the making of small fibers that assist the migration of newborn neurons (Saghatelyan, 2004). Many neurotransmitters—including dopamine, serotonin, acetylcholine, and glutamate—have been implicated in stimulating adult neurogenesis (Kempermann, 2002).

Environmental stimuli can greatly affect the proliferation and survival of newborn neurons in the adult CNS. Exposure of rodents to an *enriched (complicated) environment* increases neurogenesis and promotes nerve cell survival (Brown, 2003; Kempermann, 1997; Nilsson et al., 1999). *Physical exercise*, such as running, promotes neurogenesis by increasing cell proliferation and survival of the new neurons in rodents (van Praag, 1999a, 1999b, 2002). Vascular endothelial growth factor (VEGF) signaling may be responsible for the increased neurogenesis by both enriched environment and running (Cao, 2004; Fabel, 2003). Hippocampus-dependent learning, such as blink reflex or water maze learning, appears to increase the survival of new neurons that have been generated only at a particular time window before the training (Gould, 1999a; Leuner, 2004; van Praag, 1999a).

Interestingly, adult neurogenesis is also regulated by psychotropic drugs (Duman, 2001; Fuchs, 2000). Long-term administration of different classes of antidepressants, including serotonin and norepinephrine-selective reuptake inhibitors, increases adult neurogenesis, likely due to increasing synaptic transmission and subsequent increased nerve electrical impulse formation.

Studies have shown that several drugs of abuse, such as stimulants and opiates, decrease neurogenesis and nerve cell migration, and increase cell death rates (Eisch, 2000, 2006). Alcohol intoxication also decreases neurogenesis by inhibiting cell proliferation, migration and newborn cell survival (Crews 2003, 2008). Some of the inhibitory effects of substances of abuse on neurogenesis are likely, at least in part, due to the fact that these substances increase circulating CRF and cortisol.

Rewiring Brain Networks

Reversibility of alcohol- and drug-related cognitive function also may be the result of "neuroplastic" reorganization of key brain-cell networks. Some researchers have proposed that such reorganization may contribute to the success of alcoholism treatment. Using advanced imaging techniques, Pfefferbaum and colleagues (2001) examined the brain activity of cognitively impaired alcoholic participants during a series of tests designed to assess cognitive function. They found that although the alcoholic subjects had abnormal patterns of brain activation, compared with control subjects, they were able to complete the tasks equally well, suggesting that the brain systems in alcoholics can be functionally reorganized so that tasks formerly performed by alcohol-damaged brain systems are shunted to alternative brain systems. This finding—that cognitively impaired alcoholic patients use different brain pathways from unimpaired patients to achieve equivalent outcomes—also was suggested in a study of patients in Twelve-Step treatment programs (Mortgenstern, 1999). Functional brain reorganization may be particularly advantageous for adolescent alcohol abusers in treatment, because their developing brains are still in the process of establishing nerve-cell networks (Spear, 2000).

Brain Cell Regeneration

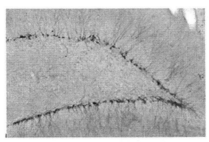

Chronic ethanol ingestion

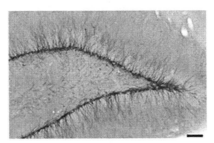

**Chronic ethanol ingestion
followed by14-days abstinence**

The above picture shows the effects of neurogenesis and neuroplasticity in a slice of a rodent brain during abstinence following chronic alcohol ingestion. The images show slides of brain cortex in chronic ethanol ingestion (top picture) and after 14 days of abstinence (bottom picture). Note the prominent increase in new neurons and their branches (exhibited by dark staining) being formed after 2 weeks of abstinence in the lower picture (Reproduced with permission from Nixon and Crews, 2004).

Brain growth has been observed not only in the recovering addict and alcoholic, but also in individuals performing specific physical or cognitive tasks. MRI studies have shown growth in the cerebellum (back of the brain used in coordination) in jugglers (Draganski, 2004; Driemeyer, 2008), the hippocampus in medical students studying for exams (Draganski, 2006), and the frontal and temporal lobes in meditators (Holzel, 2011). Interestingly, the amygdala has been shown to decrease in size in individuals under severe stress when stressors are removed (Holzel, 2010). Indeed, the adult brain exhibits substantial plasticity in response to change and gives us all hope in improving our cognitive and emotional health in the future.

Stress Inhibits Neurogenesis

Both physical and psychosocial stress paradigms, as well as some animal models of depression, lead to a decrease in cell proliferation in the brain (Duman, 2001; Fuchs, 2000). *This decrease results from the activation of the hypothalamic pituitary-adrenal axis, which is known to inhibit adult neurogenesis* (Cameron, 1994). Both structure and function of the hippocampus are altered by stress. Several studies have shown that increasing levels of corticosteroids cause atrophy, inhibit adult neurogenesis, and impair hippocampus-dependent learning. Other studies have shown that adverse experience limited to early life, specifically removal of rat pups from their mother for three hours each day, decreases production of new granule neurons in adulthood through a corticosteroid-dependent mechanism. The authors indicate that the impaired neurogenesis persists into adulthood, which may contribute to human adult depression (Kempermann, 2002; Ming, 2005). Similar impairments in hippocampal neurogenesis have been reproduced in adult rodents and primates subject to inescapable stress (Shors, 2001; Gould, 1997, 1998; Lemaire, 2000; Kozorovitsky, 2004). Cortisol reduces neurogenesis in the SGZ (Cameron, 1994, 1999). Reducing corticosteroid levels in aged rats can restore the rate of cell proliferation, which suggests that aged neural progenitors retain their proliferation capacity as in younger adult animals (Cameron, 1999). Other hormones, including estrogen and prolactin, have been shown to promote adult neurogenesis. (The girls win again!)

Summary

There are large volumes of data showing cognitive impairment in addiction. Impairment is most apparent in decision-making ability and consequently, in interoception and other higher executive functions. Memory is consistently impaired with addiction. The degree of impairment depends upon the drug of choice and degree of abuse. Nearly all drugs of abuse act directly on nervous function, however, addiction-related cortisol elevations have been shown to magnify addiction-related impairment. Stress itself causes cognitive impairment. Cognitive impairment contributes to continued compulsive drug use despite negative consequences. Addiction-related cognitive impairment is at least partially reversible due to continued neurogenesis and neuroplasticity in adulthood.

BOOK II

Recovering Stolen Goods

Chapter 7

Twelve-Step Recovery: Reducing Fear, Anger, and Stress

'I am a grateful alcoholic. For sixteen years, I have had the gift of participating in this program, working the steps and getting the daily reprieve from the obsession to drink. Most of all, I can say that I have peace of mind . . . . peace in my heart.'
~To paraphrase Jane S., Alcoholics Anonymous member celebrating sixteen years of sobriety at an AA meeting in California, 2009.

Experience, Strength, and Hope

Sixteen years of sobriety to any active alcoholic or addict seems like an eternity, if not entirely impossible. The woman quoted above is a successful, fortyish businesswoman, a wife and mother in South Orange County, California. She further shared her *"experience, strength and hope"* in the AA meeting, attended by about thirty recovering members, about how she got sober and stayed sober. She shared that she works the Twelve Steps in their entirety every \three years or so, goes to a meeting at least four times a week, has a sponsor, and is of service to other alcoholics. Every morning she turns her life and will over to her Higher Power (who happens to be the God of her understanding) meditates every morning and every night, and does a personal tenth step at the close of her day. She emphasized that her sobriety was a daily gift based on a fit *spiritual condition* with a life based on honesty, acceptance, tolerance, patience, gratitude, and service to others. She was calm, centered, and dignified. She thanked Alcoholics Anonymous, the group present that evening, her family, her co-workers, and her Higher Power for her sobriety and the quality of life she has today.

Sixteen years ago, this same woman was drunk daily, separated from her family, filing for Chapter 11 bankruptcy, and was certain she was going to die an ugly, lonely alcoholic death. At that AA meeting, Jane S received a large coin. On one side was inscribed *"16"* for sixteen years of sobriety and on the other the three axioms of AA, one inscribed on each of the three sides of the AA triangle, *"unity, service, recovery."* She received a long, warm applause from the affectionate group, congratulating her on her sobriety milestone. Many hugged her after the meeting.

Stories similar to Jane S.'s are repeated across the country and the world every day. I, personally, have heard hundreds of them. They give me hope that there is recovery from my incurable disease. *There is no cure for the changes that have occurred in the deep recesses of my brain: My reward centers and related brain structures are permanently altered, sensitized to the effects of alcohol and other mood-altering drugs. I know that I am truly an alcoholic, an individual who, once I pick up a single drink, is unable to control the craving and deafening obsession to drink more and more.*

Abstinence, in and of itself, is not particularly appealing to me or most alcoholics. (I know: I loved to drink. I needed *to drink.)* True sobriety, I have learned, is not so much about not drinking or drugging, it is about developing an attitude and lifestyle that brings sufficient serenity and personal reward that drinking, or taking any mood-altering drug, is simply unnecessary.

About Twelve-Step Programs

AA's Twelve Steps are a group of principles, spiritual in their nature, which, if practiced as a way of life, can expel the obsession to drink and enable the sufferer to become happily and usefully whole.
~AA Twelve Steps and Twelve Traditions, p. 15

I was initially suspicious, even dumbfounded, by the notion that a spiritual solution was the panacea to an organic brain disease. Sure, I was most definitely an alcoholic, but I was also a scientist and a doctor. My medical practice was based on sound, empiric data, and it worked. *What was undeniable to me, however, was the observation that Alcoholics Anonymous worked for thousands, if not millions, of alcoholics before me, dating back to the 1930's. They were sober and, most remarkably, they seemed happy. In fact, if you ask an old-timer in the program, "How does it work?" the usual reply is, "Real good."*

There are several large studies by respectable organizations concluding the same. With the understanding that neither my sponsor, large treatment centers, AA as a whole, nor I, had a reasonable explanation of how a spiritual awakening could heal an organic brain disease, I needed a lot of encouragement. Faith was not natural to me. I needed lots of encouragement and, better still, *proof.* Seeing the challenge I presented to my sponsor, he opened up his *Big Book* (basic text of Alcoholics Anonymous, 1939) and showed me *"The Promises."* He said, "Do the work and this is what you'll get . . . ."

The *Big Book of Alcoholics Anonymous* makes twelve promises to those who work the steps and follow the principles and practices of the program. After describing the Twelve Steps and the rather extraordinary amount of work they entail, the authors of the *Big Book* give us the payoff, the reward for all this work. In AA, we call the reward *"The Promises."* According to the *Big Book,*

> *"If we are painstaking about this phase of our development (working the steps), we will be amazed before we are half way through . . .*

1. *We are going to know a new freedom and a new happiness.*
2. *We will not regret the past nor wish to shut the door on it.*
3. *We will comprehend the word serenity.*
4. *We will know peace.*
5. *No matter how far down the scale we have gone, we will see how our experience can benefit others.*
6. *That feeling of uselessness and self-pity will disappear.*
7. *We will lose interest in selfish things and gain interest in our fellows.*
8. *Self-seeking will slip away.*
9. *Our whole attitude and outlook upon life will change.*

10. *Fear of people and of economic insecurity will leave us.*

11. *We will intuitively know how to handle situations which used to baffle us.*

12. *We will suddenly realize that God is doing for us what we could not do for ourselves.*

Are these extravagant promises? We think not. They are being fulfilled among us—sometimes quickly, sometimes slowly. They will always materialize if we work for them."

~ "The Promises," *Big Book*, pp. 83-84.

Now the program had my attention. There was a bigger payoff to getting sober than getting my family back and placating my professional associations: inner peace, freedom, happiness, intuition, and alleviation of fear. I was excited. In the months to follow, I undertook the program with enthusiasm.

I got a sponsor and worked the steps, meditated daily, read the *Big Book* and the *Twelve Steps and Twelve Traditions* and went to lots of meetings. Today, I am sober, too. Although I have good days and bad days, I can honestly say that, overall, I am reasonably happy, at least content. One thing for sure, having worked the steps, my stress level has been cut in half. Rather than react with fear or anger to every little indiscretion of my family or co-workers, blip in the stock market, traffic jam, or most recently, when a neighbor's dog pooped on my front lawn and left it. I have learned to take these things in stride. I *"let it go"* and *"turn it over,"* in AA terminology. In my drinking days, these things used to infuriate me. (I'd be lying if I didn't tell you the dog poop didn't irritate me a bit.) This reminds me of a definition of "stress" I heard one day in an AA meeting: *Stress: noun. def: "That feeling you get when you can't beat the sh— out of someone who desperately deserves it."* A.k.a, a "poop-ectomy?" (joking, please)

Of course, a physical "poop-ectomy" of the dog owner is not a realistic solution to the poop on the lawn problem. Finding the responsible neighbor could take weeks of surveillance and money lost to hidden cameras and the like. The legal fees for the "poop-ectomy" would be enormous. The program tells us to pray that neighbor gets all the things in life that I would want for myself. I know many AA members that can do this. Sometimes I can, and sometimes I cannot. The program also teaches us to say to ourselves, "The person who did that to me is sick and I hope and pray he gets better, for his own sake." The latter approach comes more easily to me. I believe the person who can do the first approach has better recovery than I do. *The important thing is not to be angry and stressed over any event, regardless of its significance. Recovering people never beat the poop out of anything or anybody, including themselves.* (By the way, I picked up the poop, said a quick prayer of forgiveness for the neighbor, and went on to have a great day.)

In recovery, I practice the spiritual principles of patience, tolerance, and acceptance in all my affairs. In return, I am no longer constantly experiencing friction with the world around me. My stress level is manageable. I have relative peace in my mind, can focus on my work and my family, have a normal blood pressure (without meds), eat modestly, enjoy my hobbies, and sleep well at night. No doubt, my cortisol levels are relatively low. For this, I am grateful to the Twelve-Step program of Alcoholics Anonymous.

My sponsor and I agree that I have more work to do. Indeed the *Big Book* says we get but a *"daily reprieve based on a fit spiritual condition."* The program emphasizes *daily*, not weekly, monthly, or yearly. Achieving and maintaining that condition takes a daily commitment and work. The notion of working for happiness is not what the alcoholic or addict, like me, wants to hear. On a bad day, I could say, "Darn it. I'm an alcoholic. I don't like what's going on in my life. I want a quick fix. I want it now and I want it when I want it." Certainly, if not said, these are the thoughts in my alcoholic mind.

My sponsor is quick to remind me that the last time I picked up a drink I could not stop, and came within a millimeter of losing my family, my career, and my life! When I am having a bad day, my sponsor will exercise the sponsor's prerogative and preach a bit: *"Lou, let's try the AA way . . . The effect might not be instantaneous, but it won't kill you or get you thrown in jail either. You might even get to like it . . . . I did."* After some time and hard work, I did, too. *"It works if you work it,"* is another old AA slogan. (AA has a number of catchy slogans coined by recovering alcoholics, young and old, since the 1930's, which are terrific.)

The *Big Book* recognizes the struggles of the alcoholic like me. It reads, *"No one among us has been able to maintain anything like perfect adherence to these principles. We are not saints. The point is that we are willing to grow along spiritual lines. We claim spiritual progress rather than spiritual perfection."* (*AA Big Book*, p. 60) In summary: On good days, I am happy and stress free. On bad days, I have manageable stress and, as long as I work the program, I have hope of getting re-centered and able to cope. *On ALL days, I don't need to drink; I don't want to drink.*

A Twelve-Step program is a set of guiding principles outlining a course of action for recovery from addiction, compulsion, or other behavioral problems. Twelve-Step methods have been adopted to address a wide range of substance abuse and dependency problems. Over two hundred self-help organizations—often known as fellowships, with a worldwide membership of millions—now employ Twelve-Step principles for recovery. Narcotics Anonymous was formed by addicts who did not relate to the specifics of alcohol dependency. Similar demographic preferences related to the addict's drug of choice have led to the creation of Cocaine Anonymous, Crystal Meth Anonymous, Pills Anonymous and Marijuana Anonymous, to name a few. Behavioral issues—such as compulsion for, and/or addiction to, gambling, food, sex, hoarding, debiting and work—are addressed in Twelve-Step fellowships. Auxiliary groups such as Al-Anon and Nar-Anon—for friends and family members of alcoholics and addicts, respectively—help the co-dependent family member of the addict or alcoholic recover from being "addicted to the addict."

Why Anonymous?

Alcoholics Anonymous (AA) was the first Twelve-Step fellowship, founded in 1935 by Bill Wilson and Dr. Bob Smith, known to AA members as "Bill W" and "Dr. Bob," in Akron, Ohio. They established the tradition within the *"anonymous"* Twelve-Step programs of using only first names due to the popular perception at the time that alcoholics suffered from a moral failing. Anonymity has a strong tradition in Twelve-Step recovery groups. In my opinion, *anonymity protects the members from the stress of being judged* by individuals not empathetic or sympathetic to their illness or its accompanying problems.

For example, when I share my story or my woes in a room of alcoholics, I feel good. I am not anxious or stressed. We collectively laugh at the funny parts and mourn the sad. However, when I share my story with a non-alcoholic (we call these people "normies"), I feel embarrassed, anxious, and stressed. Given that reducing stress is key to recovery, anonymity is crucial to the healing process.

Originally proposed by Alcoholics Anonymous (AA) as a method of recovery from alcoholism, the *Twelve Steps* were first published in the book, *Alcoholics Anonymous: The Story of How More Than One Hundred Men Have Recovered From Alcoholism* in 1939. The book would later be referred to as the *"Big Book."*

A Physical, Mental, and Spiritual Malady

In the Twelve-Step recovery program, addiction is described as a disease of three dimensions: physical, mental, and spiritual. The three-dimensional model proposed in Twelve-Step programs was not intended to be a scientific explanation; it is only a perspective that Twelve-Step organizations have found useful.

For addicts and alcoholics, the physical dimension is described by the program as an *"allergy-like" bodily reaction* (an abnormal reaction to a common substance) resulting in the compulsion to continue using substances after the initial use. The statement in the First Step that the individual is "powerless" over the substance-abuse related behavior at issue refers to the lack of control over this compulsion, which persists despite any negative consequences that may be endured as a result. As we discussed in Chapter 4, due to neural sensitization, the alcoholic and addict receive powerful reward center activation when exposed to mood-altering substances. The addict, therefore, is compelled by exaggerated limbic activity to ingest more and more of their drug of choice.

The programs refer to a *"mental obsession,"* described as the cognitive processes that cause the individual to repeat the compulsive behavior after some period of abstinence, either knowing that the result will be an inability to stop or operating under the delusion that the result will be different. The description in the First Step of the life of the alcoholic or addict as *"unmanageable"* refers, in part, to the lack of choice that the mind of the addict or alcoholic has acquired concerning whether to drink or use again. We have learned in previous chapters that the cravings of an addict, centered in and around the limbic system, are strong in response to specific cues and are magnified with stress.

Twelve-Step groups refer to the disease of addiction in the spiritual dimension as a *"spiritual malady."* Spiritual maladies cause emotional distress, or stress. Per Twelve-Step programs, spiritual maladies are numerous, and include dishonesty, resentment, fear, and guilt (from harm to others). Spiritual maladies are considered to be rooted in *"self-centeredness,"* a primary character defect.

The process of working the steps is intended to replace self-centeredness With <u>selflessness</u>, a spiritual attribute conducive to improving interpersonal relationships, encouraging altruism and empathy, and, most importantly, <u>reducing stress</u>. Working the steps involves taking personal inventory of fears, resentments and character defects, all of which contribute to stress in the addict or alcoholic.

Recovering members are taught to *"turn over"* their fears, resentments and guilt to a Higher Power, be it God, the group, a constellation of stars, or whatever. Twelve-Step participants are encouraged to live a life of service and gratitude. In Twelve-Step groups, this is known as a *"spiritual awakening."* This should not be confused with abreaction, which produces dramatic, but ephemeral changes. In Twelve-Step fellowships, "spiritual awakening" is believed to develop, most frequently, slowly over a period of time.

> *"The terms "spiritual experience" and "spiritual awakening" are used many times in this book (AA Big Book) which, upon careful reading shows that the personality change sufficient to bring about recovery from alcoholism (addiction) has manifested itself among us in many difference forms."*
> -*AA Big Book*, Appendix II, p. 567.

Twelve-Step Meetings and Sponsors

It is suggested that members regularly attend meetings with other members who share their particular recovery problem. There are thousands of Twelve Step groups around the country with meeting times from dawn until late in the evening. Regular Twelve-Step group members attend at least one meeting a week and frequently five or more. The meeting is a forum for members to share their challenges with addiction as well as life in general. Meetings provide empathetic support for the members. Members are encouraged to get a "home group" where other members get to know you and your life circumstances. The price is right: meetings are free. A basket is passed for the Seventh Tradition donations, typically a dollar per member per meeting, if they can afford it, which pays for rent, coffee, literature, etc. "Meeting makers make it," as the old AA slogan goes. The theory behind why attendance at meetings and participation in the group promotes sobriety is covered in depth in Chapter 9.

Members are also encouraged to get a sponsor. Sponsors share their experience, strength, and hope with their sponsees. A sponsor is not a therapist offering professional advice. A sponsor is simply another alcoholic or addict in recovery who is willing to share his or her journey through the Twelve Steps. Sponsors and sponsees participate in activities that lead to spiritual growth. These may include practices such as literature discussion and study, meditation, and journaling. Completing the Twelve Steps and having a solid recovery foundation are the usual prerequisites of a sponsor. Sponsors guide the newcomers, the sponsees, though the Steps. Sponsees typically do their Fifth Step—a review of a moral inventory of fears, resentments, and harms, written in the format described in the *Big Book* under the Fourth Step—with their sponsor. The Fifth Step (moral inventory), as well as the Ninth Step (making amends for prior harms), have been compared to confession and penitence. *Many philosophers, religious writers and psychologists have recognized AA's practices, noting that such practices produce intrinsic modifications in the person —exonerating, redeeming, and purifying them. It unburdens them of their wrongs, liberates them, and, for some, promises their salvation.*

Effectiveness of Twelve-Step Programs

While research into Twelve-Step approaches began in the 1940s, following AA's founding in the thirties, the breadth and depth of research increased in the eighties and particularly the nineties. This resulted in research of improved methodological quality into both the benefits of Twelve Step programs as well AA/Twelve-Step involvement per se. Coupled with positive research outcomes, the overall confidence in AA's effectiveness grew, along with interest in facilitating connections between treatment programs and Twelve-Step groups. In addition, the growth of managed health care reduced the length and intensity of professional addictions treatment (Humphreys et al, 1997), increasing the pressure for cost effective treatment approaches. In the addiction literature, Twelve-Step programs are referred to as belonging to the Twelve-Step Facilitation (TSF) model of addiction treatment.

TSF models are inexpensive to implement, and Twelve-Step and other self-help groups are ubiquitous and basically free, making TSF an attractive option. Anyone can start a Twelve-Step group by contacting the general service counsel of the organization of their interest, finding a meeting place (sometimes a person's home) and adopting a readily available meeting protocol.

A body of continually developing research now supports TSF treatment for addiction and alcoholism. In 2001, a workgroup of national experts on substance abuse was convened by the Center for Substance Abuse Treatment (CSAT) and the Veterans Health Administration (VHA) to examine evidence on the effectiveness of drug and alcohol self-help groups. Findings, including implications for the field, were subsequently published (Humphreys et al, 2004). The report concluded that:

"A significant body of research has documented an association between Twelve-Step self-help group participation and positive outcomes and has suggested mechanisms by which these positive outcomes are generated. In addition, millions of Americans have 'voted with their feet' by participating in addiction related self-help groups, sometimes in the face of ambivalence by clinicians. Many improvements remain to be made in self-help group research, but at present the following represent reasonable conclusions based on the existing research: Longitudinal studies associate Alcoholics Anonymous and Narcotics Anonymous participation with greater likelihood of abstinence, improved social functioning, and greater self-efficacy. Participation seems more helpful when members engage in other group activities in addition to attending meetings; Twelve-Step groups significantly reduce health care utilization and costs, removing a significant burden from the health care system; Self-help groups are best viewed as a form of continuing care rather than as a substitute for acute treatment services; and, Randomized trials with coerced populations suggest that AA combined with professional treatment is superior to AA alone."

Donovan (2007, 2008) presents additional key points derived from research into Twelve-Step involvement: Longitudinal studies usually find that Twelve-Step involvement after treatment is associated with higher rates of abstinence regardless of the kind of treatment received. Consistent and early attendance/involvement leads to better substance use outcomes. *Attendance is not, in itself, involvement.* When AA attendance and AA involvement (e.g. reading Twelve-Step literature, getting a sponsor, "working" the steps, or helping set up meetings) are both measured, involvement is a stronger predictor of outcome; Even small amounts of participation may be helpful in increasing abstinence, whereas higher doses may be needed to reduce relapse intensity.

Kaskutas (2009) recently conducted a review of the literature on AA effectiveness. She concluded, "The evidence for AA effectiveness is strong" for five of the six study criteria she examined, with conclusions uncertain regarding the sixth.

"Get a sponsor." "Be of service." "Use the telephone." "Work the steps." These oft-repeated suggestions are familiar to anyone who has attended Twelve-Step meetings, where getting active is considered recovery's key. That is the main goal of all Twelve Step Facilitation (TSF) therapy models: to encourage not only attendance, but also *active involvement* in Twelve-Step groups and activities. While research suggests attendance is a precursor to involvement in Twelve-Step groups, multiple studies indicate that active involvement is a better predictor of positive outcomes. Donovan and Floyd go on to document research that demonstrates that early involvement in Twelve-Step activities (during treatment) yields better results, and that engagement is a better predictor of positive results than attendance. Project MATCH is the most well known study of the effectiveness of Twelve-Step groups and TSF and the one study with the greatest weight of supporting follow-up research.

Project MATCH was the largest alcohol treatment research trial ever done, involving more than 1,700 alcohol-dependent patients studied over time in nine clinical research sites across the United States (Project MATCH Research Group, 1993, 1997, 1998). Project MATCH included two independent study arms, one with outpatients (n = 952), the other with patients in aftercare following inpatient treatment (n = 774). All participants were randomly assigned to TSF, Cognitive-Behavioral Therapy (CBT), or Motivational Enhancement Therapy (MET). Participants received a twelve-week intervention, a one-year follow-up and, for those in the outpatient arm, two three-year follow-ups. While the goal was to study the matching of patients to a specific treatment intervention, the most significant findings lay in the comparative effectiveness of the several interventions. Highlights related to TSF include the following:

- At one- and three-year follow-ups, TSF was found to be comparable in effectiveness to CBT and MET (Project MATCH 1997). Patients in all three conditions improved significantly in drinking-related, psychological, and life-functioning outcomes.

- TSF was more effective than CBT or MET in promoting abstinence among outpatients (For example, at the three-year follow-up, 36 percent of TSF patients reported being abstinent for the previous three months, compared with about 24 percent in CBT and 27 percent in MET conditions ($p < 0.007$) (Project MATCH 1998).
- TSF was significantly more effective than either CBT or MET in increasing AA active participation, as marked by the frequency of attending meetings, having and serving as a sponsor, following the twelve steps, and considering oneself an AA member (Tonigan et al. 2003).
- AA participation positively predicted the frequency of abstinent days in the post-treatment period (Connors et al. 2001).
- Of the twenty-one client attributes, two were the most powerful predictors of long-term abstinence outcome: (1) readiness to change and (2) self-efficacy (clients' confidence in their ability to abstain).
- Among clients with social networks supportive of drinking, AA involvement was higher for TSF clients (62 percent) than for those receiving MET (38 percent) or CBT (25 percent) (Longabaugh 1998).

The Project MATCH TSF model sought to facilitate two general goals in individuals with alcohol or other drug problems: (1) acceptance, or the need for abstinence, from alcohol or other drug use; and (2) surrender, or the willingness to participate actively in Twelve-Step fellowships as a means of sustaining sobriety. These main goals were then broken down into a series of cognitive, emotional, relationship, behavioral, social, and spiritual objectives.

A study that resembled Project MATCH enrolled 3,018 male military veterans with substance-use disorders across fifteen program sites (Ouimette, 1997, 1998). Drug dependence was not excluded, and 51 percent of the men had co-occurring alcohol and drug dependence. Participants received inpatient detoxification, followed by twenty-one to twenty-eight days of intensive Twelve-Step treatment, CBT, or both. Alcohol and drug abuse declined equally in all three groups, and subjects were referred for outpatient aftercare and self-help groups. After one year, involvement in a Twelve-Step group predicted better outcome, regardless of the initial treatment.

Unlike earlier studies, this trial found that individuals with co-occurring psychiatric disorders and those legally mandated to get treatment did as well at one-year follow-up as those without these variables. It provides additional evidence that Twelve-Step treatments can reduce substance use across varied populations, including patients with co-occurring alcohol and drug dependence.

Another widely quoted study focused on outcomes of the Minnesota Model treatment, as delivered at Hazelden in Center City, Minnesota (Stinchfield and Owen, 1998). Stinchfield and Owen collected data on 1,083 men and women at four points: when they entered treatment at Hazelden, and at one month, six months, and twelve months after treatment. Three major findings were reported:

- At the twelve-month point, 53 percent of these people said that they had abstained from alcohol and other drugs during the year after treatment.
- Another 35 percent said that they had reduced their chemical use.
- Between 70 and 90 percent of these clients also reported improved quality of life in areas, such as family relationships and job performance.

These results, consistent with other studies of the Minnesota Model treatment, compare favorably with outcomes reported for other private treatment programs, such as the Betty Ford Center, Talbot, and Sierra Tucson. The Minnesota Model, with a Twelve-Step foundation, fuses many elements: a residential setting, group therapy, individual counseling, lectures, discussions, assignments, attendance at Twelve Step meetings, and more. And as part of the model, clients receive services from a team of counselors, nurses, physicians, psychologists, recreational therapists, and spiritual care specialists. Treatment is individualized, and aspects of Cognitive Behavioral and Motivational Enhancement Therapy are woven in.

According to Hazelden, what unifies these disparate elements is the Twelve Step philosophy: lifelong abstinence is the goal of recovery, and frequent attendance at Twelve Step meetings is the primary way to maintain abstinence over the long term. Stinchfield and Owen (1998) put it this way: *"The primary agent of change is group affiliation and practicing behaviors consistent with the Twelve-Step program of AA."*

Taking the Mystery Out of the Miracle of Twelve-Step Recovery

> *"(Having worked the steps) . . . we have ceased fighting anything or anyone—even alcohol! For by this time sanity will have returned. We will seldom be interested in liquor (our addiction). If tempted, we recoil from it as from a hot flame . . . This is the miracle of it. We are not fighting it, neither are we avoiding temptation. We feel as though we have been placed in a position of neutrality—safe and protected."*
>
> *~AA Big Book*, pp. 84-85

When I see the word "fight," I see the word "stress." As discussed in Chapter 5, the stress response or "fight-or-flight" response is characterized by physiological changes in our bodies that make us feel uncomfortable. *When we feel fear or anger, or both, the addict or alcoholic feels a need to medicate with drugs or alcohol.* The "fight-or-flight" response is fundamental to our survival and was first described in animal species. In the ancient evolutionary environment, when an animal or early man was faced with the "stress" of a predator, or a mating or foraging opponent, one had three options: fight, flee, or die (do not reproduce or eat). Our adrenaline surges, blood pressure rises, blood flow to muscles increases and to our intestines decreases, and our stress hormone, cortisol, surges, releasing sugar from our liver and muscles. Stress is the most prevalent cause of relapse in the recovering addict and a predominant predisposing factor in the development of addiction.

"Fight or flight" may be rephrased for the modern man as "anger and fear." Indeed, "stress" has many descriptors: fight, anger, resentment, bitterness, frustration, fear, anxiety and worry. In the *Big Book of Alcoholics Anonymous* the words "fight" or "fighting" are mentioned ten times, "resentment, anger, frustration or bitterness" seventy times and "fear, anxiety, or worry" seventy-six times. Less potent forms of emotional stress are also mentioned: "guilt," six times, and "remorse," eight times. *Thus, "stress" in its many faces is mentioned in the Big Book 170 times.* The authors of the *Big Book* were well aware of how important it was to reduce stress in the alcoholic seeking recovery.

The Twelve-Steps were designed to establish abstinence from drinking alcohol, but clearly, the authors had insight into the fact that abstinence was not sustainable unless the recovering alcoholic was given tools to manage life's stressors. The Twelve Steps are the framework of these tools. Sobriety is not just about abstinence from drinking and drugging. Sobriety encompasses an attitude of living that obviates the use of mood-altering substances of any sort. In the *Big Book* chapter titled *"How it Works"* it states; *"Our liquor was but a symptom (of our disease). We had to get down to the root causes and conditions."* (*AA Big Book*, p. 64) The book then asks readers to start their fourth-step personal inventory of fears, resentments, and harms (guilt).

Working the Twelve Steps: Reducing Fear, Anger, and Stress

These are the original Twelve Steps as published by Alcoholics Anonymous in 1939:

1. *We admitted we were powerless over alcohol (or our addiction)-that our lives had become unmanageable.*
2. *Came to believe that a Power greater than ourselves could restore us to sanity.*
3. *Made a decision to turn our will and our lives over to the care of God as we understood Him.*
4. *Made a searching and fearless moral inventory of ourselves.*
5. *Admitted to God, to ourselves, and to another human being the exact nature of our wrongs.*
6. *Were entirely ready to have God remove all these defects of character.*
7. *Humbly asked Him to remove our shortcomings.*
8. *Made a list of all persons we had harmed, and became willing to make amends to them all.*
9. *Made direct amends to such people wherever possible, except when to do so would injure them or others.*
10. *Continued to take personal inventory and when we were wrong promptly admitted it.*
11. *Sought through prayer and meditation to improve our conscious contact with God, as we understood Him, praying only for knowledge of His will for us and the power to carry that out.*

12. Having had a spiritual awakening as the result of these steps, we tried to carry this message to alcoholics, and to practice these principles in all our affairs.

Step 1. We admitted we were powerless over alcohol (or our addiction)-that our lives had become unmanageable.

Step 1 is an admission of powerlessness. The writings of AA tell us that victory over alcohol is only possible if we first admit complete defeat. Although counterintuitive at first glance, upon further reflection one can see that admitting complete defeat is a recognition that old lifestyle choices were not working and, certainly, the use of alcohol or drugs was not working. By admitting defeat and powerlessness we clear the path, going forward, for a new approach to life.

The First Step begins with admitting powerlessness over alcohol or other drugs, but its application is expanded in the *Big Book* to apply to all of life's twists and turns. In my active addiction to alcohol, there was no doubt that I was powerless over its effect on me. *Once I took a single drink, my brain's limbic reward centers would light up like a Roman candle while, concurrently, my cortisol levels would go up and my decision-making centers in my frontal lobe would shut down.* The first drink lead to a second, and a third, and a . . . whatever . . . until I passed out. I was literally crippled by a single drink of a two-carbon sugar; therefore, admitting powerlessness over alcohol was not difficult.

As an educated professional and control freak, admitting powerlessness over the rest of life, however, was something else entirely. I would say to myself, "Don't you know who I am? How hard I work? All that I've accomplished? I'm the go-to guy . . ." and all that absolutely pathetic, arrogant nonsense. My counselor at Betty Ford, a big guy in his sixties who used to be an offensive tackle for the Chicago Bears, aptly remarked one day, as he looked down at me though his bifocals, chuckling a bit, "You doctors are the worst . . . geesh! . . . when it comes to accepting powerlessness over life," its unpredictability and often unforeseen hardships. He found us MD's rather humorous. He called us "MDeities" sometimes to really rub it in, as he ramped up his deep chuckle. "You sure earned your chair here in the treatment center, Doc . . ." Very funny.

The *Big Book* refers to the active alcoholic as an actor on a stage, forever and futilely trying to run the whole show. If things would only go his way, life would be good, he would be happy. More often than not, the show does not come off the way that suits him. In reaction to this, he becomes angry, indignant and self-pitying. He is in friction with his world; he is stressed. Admitting that he does not run the show is the first step in removing this stress.

The First Step is usually taken after the active alcoholic or addict has reached bottom. It is said tongue-in-cheek in the halls of Alcoholics Anonymous: "Nobody walks through these doors because they're having a great day." My bottom was my family giving me an ultimatum: "Sober up or get out." My bottom was my licensing board telling me (and I paraphrase): "Sober up, don't drink at all, get drug tested, or don't practice medicine in this state . . ." Ouch! They were right. My bottom was looking in the mirror and seeing a bloated, desperate man who only barely resembled his true self. My bottom was almost dying twice in the last weeks of my final run of rampant debauchery. The purists of the 'reward-punishment' and 'pleasure-pain' motivational models of human behavior could say that the pleasure I was receiving from drinking alcohol was now finally eclipsed by the pain in continuing to drink. They were correct. I hit bottom.

But the problem was only partially mitigated by my putting down the bottle. The majority of the problem was deeply ingrained in my personality and my controlling, all-powerful attitude. The sobering facts were that, according to my plan, I was out of work for a minimum of three to six months, my finances were tanking, I was holding onto a once-thriving medical career by a thread, and I was holding onto a family—and, arguably, my life—by a thread. My life was unmanageable, to say the least.

The admission of powerlessness is, however, quite liberating and brings a sense of calm to the addict or alcoholic (BP and stress hormones notch down a bit). The writers of the *Big Book*, as usual, say it so well: "*When we have finally admitted without reservation that we are powerless over alcohol, we are apt to breathe a great sigh of relief, saying, 'Well, thank God that's over!'*" (Twelve Steps and Twelve Traditions, p. 73)

Thank God, indeed. *Here I was, incarcerated in a treatment center, fat and bloated, with sky-high blood pressure, stress hormones off the chart, cognitive function a fraction of normal, and emotional state in a perfect storm of fear, confusion, anger, and despair. Suicide was an option . . . but not yet.* Life was a mess, *but giving up is not what I do,* so I was going to give the program of AA a shot. I once heard *The Promises* from the *Big Book*, and how they came true for thousands before me in my predicament or worse, and I was going to give it what might have been my last effort to stay on the planet. *Step 1 was the beginning of my freedom.*

Step 2. Came to believe that a Power greater than ourselves could restore us to sanity.

Step 2 gave me hope that someone or something could restore my sanity. I believe in God, although I am not at all religious. Although raised Catholic, I abandoned the church many years ago for many reasons. I personally believe that organized religion has many benefits; however, it has shortcomings in the hands of us mortal men. So for me to turn to God in this time of crisis did not come easy. The Twelve-Step program does not require a belief in God, only a belief in a *"Power greater than myself."* (*AA Big Book*, p.47) For me, that power was perceived in the God of my understanding as well as the individuals in the program who had walked the path ahead of me. They gave me hope that I would recover. At the time, I had no clue how that would happen, but my hope was already helping reduce my stress level: I could get through the day without crying, I could focus the best I could in the groups, counseling sessions, and step work and, most nights, I could sleep more than a few hours.

Step 3. Made a decision to turn our will and our lives over to the care of God as we understood Him.

Step 2 gave me hope that someone or some program, maybe even God, could restore my sanity. In Step 3, I was asked to turn my life and will over to my Higher Power. For many of us alcoholics this is a tall order. We are selfish creatures and like being in control. But, obviously, my "being in control" got me in a treatment center and life as I knew it was in tatters, so I was willing to take this step. My sponsor told me the key was to be *"honest, open and willing"* (acronym H.O.W.) and I might get it. Taking instruction from him was part of my Step Three; he was, in part, and in effect, my Higher Power. He instructed me to read p. 417 of the *Big Book* daily. It reads:

> *And acceptance is the answer to <u>all</u> my problems today. When
> I am disturbed, it is because I find some person, place, thing, or
> situation – some fact of my life – unacceptable to me, and I can find*

> *no serenity until I accept that person, place, thing, or situation as being exactly the way it is supposed to be at this moment. Nothing, absolutely nothing happens in God's (this) world by mistake. Until I could accept my alcoholism, I could not stay sober; unless I accept life completely on life's terms, I cannot be happy. I need to concentrate not so much on what needs to be changed in the world as on what needs to be changed in me and in my attitudes.*
> ~Dr. Paul C., *AA Big Book*, Fourth Edition, p. 417

Living these words takes practice and time, at least for this alcoholic. But when I feel like I actually believe this simple message, my life is better without anything outside of myself changing. The only thing changing with this step was internal: *my attitude*. Dr. Paul C. went on to write a very popular book called *A New Pair of Glasses* in which he expounds upon the idea that looking through the "clear" lenses of *acceptance* rather than the "befogged" lenses of non-acceptance, intolerance, and perpetual friction has improved his serenity many-fold over. For me, accepting life on life's terms takes work. Some days it is not easy to do myself and I need the help of my sponsor or another AA friend to put things in perspective and "defog my glasses," so to speak. My sponsor, when I present him with a nagging problem (usually trivial, although blown out of proportion in my warped mind), invariably replies, "Lou, that's a Cadillac problem. Read page 417, and get grateful for what you have . . . *now!*" (I hear this so often I should record his voiced message on my cell phone for convenient playback.) If he feels I am not really listening, he tells me to make a gratitude list: sobriety, health, healthy family, redeemable career, few bucks in the bank, etc.

Certainly, when I adopt an attitude of acceptance, and add some gratitude for good measure, my stress level drops remarkably, and almost instantaneously. I can feel my body relax, my heart rate and blood pressure drop, and my mind clear. I am able to focus on the task at hand. *"It works, if you work it,"* as they say in AA, I agree: It really does. Heck, if I keep it up, I might even live a little longer—sober.

Step 4. Made a searching and fearless moral inventory of ourselves.

The Fourth Step requires real work, as one is instructed to create a written inventory of resentments, fears, and sexual and other harms (things we are guilty about). This step, if taken diligently, usually leads to twenty or more written pages of our problems, all of which cause stress. The pages take the form of several columns. First, we list the name of the person or thing that is causing this problem. Second, we are asked to identify what it affects: my self-esteem, financial security, relationships, etc. Third, we are asked to identify what the cause might be: selfishness, self-will, dishonesty, denial, impatience, intolerance, etc. Finally, we are asked to identify "my part" in each of the fears, resentments, etc. This last column asks us to take at least some personal responsibility for our problems.

The exercise is remarkable, if done with earnest. Quite frankly, I considered it quite a gift. I could say that if I was not an alcoholic, I would never have found AA and never been compelled to make a moral inventory of myself. My resentment list was of average length and included the usual suspects, whose names I will not divulge to protect the innocent. My sexual harms list was relatively short.

My fears list, however, was remarkably long and taught me that, basically, I lived a fear-based life. This had a powerful effect on me. The strong, self-sufficient, powerhouse doctor of my delusions was actually a frightened little boy. You name it, I feared it. I am fearful of my kids health failing. I am fearful of my wife of twenty-two years not loving me. I am fearful of losing my job. I am fearful of the markets tanking. I'm fearful of China selling a stealth bomber to North Korea and that bomber annihilating Southern California! The list goes on for many pages, but, remarkably, when I looked at the list I realized that it was really unlikely that any of these things would come true. My family and career were intact and redeemable, as long as I did not drink, and North Korea really is not my problem. One of my AA buddies referred to "fear" by the acronym: "False Evidence Appearing Real." My life was full of it. The last column, "my part," brought to my attention that many of the resentments, fears, etc. that I had were substantially of my own making. *I was responsible for causing many of them; therefore, I had power over changing them.*

Step 5. Admitted to God, to ourselves, and to another human being the exact nature of our wrongs.

As a recovering Catholic, Step 5 reminds me of the sacrament of penance, the confession of one's sins to a man, a representative of God. When I looked into this practice, I found that virtually all religions have some form of penance, contrition, absolution, or reconciliation, including Buddhism, Judaism, Christianity and Islam dating back thousands of years. The curative effect of confession has been known for centuries. Priests, ministers, and rabbis, as well as psychotherapists, attest to the universality of this human phenomenon. Dr. Carl Jung, first president of the International Psychoanalytic Association, recognized the act of confession as essential to emotional health. Simply stated, the word *confession* is an avowal of sin, made either to God or to man. When Jung referred to confession, he referred to two parts of the ritual: the need to confess and the need to be forgiven and reconciled. Through this process of confession, the confessor is relieved of stress. Jung (1961) states: "*The tremendous feeling of relief which usually follows a confession can be ascribed to the readmission of the lost sheep into the human community. His moral isolation and seclusion, which were so difficult to bear, cease. Herein lies the chief psychological value of confession.*"

Jung asserted that man is naturally religious—or better stated in the context of the current discussion, *spiritual.* According to Jung, the spiritual instinct in man is as powerful as the instinct of sex or aggression. He suggested that confessions made to the God of our understanding were an important part of the process of healing. Jung (1954) further asserts, "*Confessions made to one's secret self generally have little or no effect, whereas confessions made to another are much more promising.*" Thus, a confession is most effective when made to an empathetic and empowered human being and to the God of our understanding.

According to Jung, without confession, man remains in moral isolation. Confession is located in that place where psychology and religion meet: *guilt.* Guilt is a dominant emotion in the addict or alcoholic. The practicing addict or alcoholic does deplorable things to perpetuate their drugging and drinking. They violate laws, disregard families, and endanger innocents. The guilt I carried while practicing my disease was enormous. Confession, according to Dr. Jung, confession bridges the gap between psychology and religion. As such, Alcoholics Anonymous and Twelve Step programs bridge the gap between psychology and addiction medicine.

Dr. Jung believed that man evolved from animals. In his writings, he refers to a "*shadow,*" or our dark side. Jung (1954) states: "*The shadow represents the remnants of the beast.*" It is that which is inferior to the individual's consciousness, and that which he denies and condemns. The conscious mind, the rational mind works to conceal the shadow, banishing it to the realm of the unconscious where it is inaccessible for correction. There it lurks in the dark caves of the psyche, uncorrected and unbridled, yet distorting the performance of the conscious, rational mind. Jung (1958) states: *"Everyone carries a shadow and the less it is embodied in the individual's conscious life, the blacker and denser it is . . . . The shadow is merely somewhat inferior, primitive, maladapted and awkward, not wholly bad. It even contains childish or primitive qualities which would, in a way vitalize and embellish human existence."* Jung continues, *"The inferior and even the worthless belongs to me as my shadow and gives me substance and mass. How can I be substantial without casting a shadow? I must have a dark side too if I am to be whole; and by becoming conscious of my shadow I remember once more that I am a human being like any other."* (Jung, 1958)

I believe, at least in part, that Dr. Jung is recognizing and paying respect to primitive human instincts. During Jung's time, the neurosciences were not developed and knowledge of the full function of the limbic system and the dopamine reward pathways was just beyond theory. Today we know that the brain's reward centers generate our fundamental motivational programs. Heeding to the unbridled call of our "shadow," our limbic reward centers, our instinctual drives, can separate us from society and its norms and our personal moral code. Herein lies the roots of our fear and resentments.

Heeding to our base instincts we have sex with another's spouse, steal food or more when financially weary, or get high on drugs or alcohol when we have responsibilities that cannot be met while under the influence. When we violate our own and society's moral code, we feel guilty. We fell stressed. Guilt may be described as a form of "anger with self." Self-loathing is another form of "anger with self." *Self-loathing is stressful.* Self-pity, in contrast, is sorrow for self, usually secondary to self-centeredness. We also experience stress with sorrow. The dictionary defines sorrow as *"distress caused by loss, affliction, disappointment, etc.; grief, sadness, or regret." Self-pity is stressful.* These stress states implore us to self-medicate.

Within our limbic reward centers, particularly the amygdala, also lies our *fears*, which are usually self-centered. We fear our security will be compromised when our food, money, or other material possessions will be taken from us. We fear we will lose the love and affection of our spouses or significant others. In some circumstances, we fear we may not be able to breathe, that we may die. *Fear is stressful.*

Herein lie our *resentments*, also usually self-centered. Resentment means to "re feel" an emotion—in this reference, anger. We are angered when our spouse does not comfort us or have sex with us. We are angered when our boss does not promote us and give us more money, and we are angered when our food at the restaurant is late to the table. We are angered with ourselves for doing shameful things while intoxicated. For the alcoholic or addict, we are angry when you take our "stuff"—really angry! (My selfish, hedonistic reward centers are screaming for this stuff—don't you know!) *Resentments are stressful.* Herein lies our addiction.

As guilt, self-loathing, self-pity, fear and resentments produce stress, we have two solutions: (1) take a mood-altering substance, and risk addiction and other consequences; or (2) let go of our stress to another human being and/or our Higher Power. The *Big Book* tells us to take a pain-staking inventory of our wrongs, fears, and resentments and to share them with another empathetic human being and to God (if we have one). By doing so, the Fifth Step gives us *relief from stress.*

According to the authors of the *Big Book (p. 75)*: *"Once we have taken this step, withholding nothing, we are delighted. We can look the world in the eye. We can be alone at perfect peace and ease. Our fears fall from us. We begin to feel the nearness of our Creator. We may have had certain spiritual beliefs, but not we begin to have a spiritual experience. The feeling that the drink problem has disappeared will often come strongly."*

When I finished my Fifth Step, which took about two hours with a recovering alcoholic counselor at Betty Ford, I wanted to take a nap, not a drink. Being medically inclined, I suspect my blood pressure was low, heart rate baseline or below, and cortisol levels baseline or below. The relief was mentally and physically profound.

During the process of Step 5, the sponsor or counselor usually makes a list of character defects typifying the addict or alcoholic presenting the step. These usually include, but are not limited to: selfishness and self-centered fear, self-will (selfish, controlling behavior), dishonesty, denial (a form of dishonesty), procrastination, pride, envy, jealousy, and lethargy, to name a few. I can honestly say I had all of them to some degree or another. My most glaring defects of character were dishonesty, mostly surrounding my drinking, and selfishness, also mostly based in my drinking, but also based upon my incredible personal insecurity. Once these character defects are illuminated in Step 5, the recovering addict-alcoholic can now proceed to Steps 6 and 7.

Step 6. *Were entirely ready to have God remove all these defects of character; and Step 7. Humbly asked Him to remove our shortcomings.*

It was easy for me to take this step because I believed in God. I believe in a God that is the Creator of the universe (the deity that put the bang in the "Big Bang") and is all knowing and all powerful, and has a plan for me on this planet. I believe that God speaks to me through other men and women. I see God's message in a multitude of religious teachings and practices. I see God's message in the *Big Book of Alcoholics Anonymous*. But that is my personal belief. The authors of the *Big Book* did not want to exclude those who did not believe in God from the gifts of the program of sobriety, thus they wrote the chapter, "*We Agnostics.*" In it, the authors assert, "*If a mere code of morals or better philosophy of life were sufficient to overcome alcoholism, many of us would have recovered long ago.*" (*AA Big Book*, p. 44) The fact of the matter was, as the authors recognized, that alcohol was more powerful than any moral code or philosophy. The authors invoke the idea of "*a Power greater than ourselves,*" a "*Higher Power.*" (*AA Big Book*, p. 45) The authors go on to say that "*as soon as we were able to lay aside prejudice and express even a willingness to believe in a Power greater than ourselves, we commenced to get results, even though it was impossible for any of us to fully define or comprehend that Power, which is God. When speaking of God, we mean your own conception of God.*" (*AA Big Book*, p. 46) One can refer to a "*Creative Intelligence, a Spirit of the Universe,*" the universe itself, the breadth and depth of nature, or whatever.

Greg M. is a recovering alcoholic with four years of sobriety. He is tall, slender and handsome, and has a productive electronics business in Southern California. He is a father of a young boy. Divorced, he has a steady girlfriend. He is an atheist. I asked him how he did the steps without a "God." He told me he visualized taking a brown paper bag of crap (character defects) and flinging it into the ocean, where the waves would nudge it back to shore, but slowly, methodically, and with certainty, it would be eroded by and dispersed into the vast sea. The bag of crap would be no more.

Although I believe in God, I liked Greg's solution to ridding himself of his defects of character, fears and resentments (although I might pick a metaphor less aromatic). He realizes the importance of *letting things go as a means of reducing his stress and perpetuating his sobriety.* In his case, the "Power Greater than Himself" was the vastness and powerful consuming forces of the ocean. It could very well have been a metaphor visualizing a balloon disappearing into the vastness of the sky. The point is that we, as humans, have character flaws, fears, resentments, and guilt, and if we hold onto them, they become toxic to our emotional well-being and our relationships. Our limbic emotion centers signal fear, which signal our pituitary gland to secret corticotrophin release factor, which signals our adrenal glands to release cortisol and adrenalin. Our brains and our bodies feel stressed; we feel uncomfortable. To relieve the stress and discomfort we invoke a Power Greater than Ourselves, a Higher Power. Before entering a program of recovery, we would relieve the stress with drinking or drugging. The *Big Book* of AA clearly states the alternative of recovery: *"But when I became willing to clean house and then asked a Higher Power, God as I understood Him, to give me release (of these character defects), my obsession to drink vanished."*

Step 8. *Made a list of all persons we had harmed, and became willing to make amends to them all; and Step 9. Made direct amends to such people wherever possible, except when to do so would injure them or others.*

At first, I did not like these steps because they made me do something uncomfortable: approach someone I had harmed in some way and say that I am sorry. More so, in some cases, making amends meant being a more productive worker, or being a more attentive father or more loving spouse on a day-to-day basis. Amends made through day-to-day actions, rather than words, are what we call *"living amends."* I was hesitant. But, Dr. Jung, the authors of the *Big Book* and thousands of alcoholics before me have proven that *making amends in an effort to be free of guilt is crucial to my emotional health and my sobriety.* To make amends I had to be humble, which also did not come easily to me. But I had already begun to humble myself in Step 7, so I had a head start on humbly presenting myself to those whom I had harmed and making amends, either in words or in actions.

Initially, this step actually increased my stress level as I inventoried those who I had harmed and planned actions or penned words of amends. As I was thinking about how to approach this person, or that person, I was completely stressed out. It required courage as well as humility, and I was not sure if I had that much courage. This is where the support of my sponsor and the fellowship was critical.

I summoned the courage of several people—a movement, if you will—to get the amends process under way. After I began this process (which took several months), about half way down the list, I began to feel a great relief. People, for the most part, were open to my amends and responded favorably to them. *My guilt and shame were being alleviated, if not entirely removed. I was becoming more comfortable with myself.* With some of these people, I came closer to them and our relationships became more intimate and real. So, as stressful as it was to start, the final product was a great relief of stress with a bonus: better relationships.

Step 10. Continued to take personal inventory and when we were wrong promptly admitted it.

The *Big Book* warns us that the work of recovery is not done once we complete the Steps. According to the authors, "*It is easy to let up on the spiritual program of action and rest on our laurels. We are headed for trouble if we do, for alcohol is a subtle foe. We are not cured of alcoholism. What we really have is a daily reprieve based on a fit spiritual condition.*" (*AA Big Book*, p. 85) After the alcoholic or addict has gone through the majority of the work to clean their slate and free themselves of the stress of carrying guilt, anger and fear, now comes the daily housecleaning. Step 10 asks us to look at our day, *every* day, and take an inventory: Were we afraid, anxious, or stressed? Were we dishonest? Were we resentful? What could we do better tomorrow that we did not do today?

A friend of mine in recovery, Dr. Harry Haroutunian (2011), medical director of the Betty Ford Center Residential Treatment Program, put it this way: *"I'll take an inventory, sometimes twice a day, so it doesn't get backed up. I can't carry the debt anymore, I have to do it at noontime and during a 10th step in the evening, and make sure things are right, and if they are not right, I'll go back and try to fix them. What happened was, when I started to get that spiritual awakening and pray on a regular basis, I started to see dishonesty turn to honesty, despair turn to faith and trust, and my self-pity turn to gratitude. It was only then I began to focus back on recovery. That's the spiritual change that I was able to find."*

Noteworthy in Dr. Harry's explanation of the Tenth Step is his use of the word *"spiritual." He refers to his spiritual condition as being right with the world, being free of guilt, dishonesty, fear, resentment, self-pity (self-loathing, anger with self) and their associated stress.* Like me, Harry believes in God, however our spiritual condition is as much about being at peace with ourselves as it is about being at peace with God. It requires daily maintenance. Dr. Harry is magical.

Step 11. Sought through prayer and meditation to improve our conscious contact with God <u>as we understood Him</u>, praying only for knowledge of His will for us and the power to carry that out.

Step 11 encourages the recovering alcoholic and addict to pray and meditate on a daily basis. It is said in the circles of recovery, "Prayer is talking to God, and meditation is listening to God." In the *Big Book*, the authors mention prayer and meditation in the same paragraph as the Tenth Step inventory, asking the reader, when they retire at night, to constructively review their day, taking their Tenth Step inventory, clearing their slate, then listening to their Higher Power for guidance for tomorrow. At this time, the authors suggested a period of quiet meditation.

The practice of meditation dates back thousands of years and is practiced by numerous religious and non-religious organizations. The literature on the benefits of meditation in restoring emotional health and reducing emotional—thus, physiological—stress is immense and convincing. For this reason, I have devoted an entire chapter to the subject, Chapter 8.

Step 12. Having had a spiritual awakening as the result of these steps, we tried to carry this message to alcoholics, and to practice these principles in all our affairs.

The Twelfth Step identifies those who have done the work up to this point as having a *"spiritual awakening"* and this spiritual awakening manifests itself as a *"personality change sufficient to bring about recovery from alcoholism (addiction)."* (*AA Big Book*, p. 567) Having performed the Steps, we have begun to receive The Promises, which include freedom from fear and self-pity, serenity, peace. Alas, we are free of *stress*.

The authors of the Twelfth Step also make it clear that it is the duty of the recovering individual to share the message, the gift of recovery. Thus, altruistic works are as much a part of recovery as all the Step work before it. In the program, it is said: "To keep it, you have to give it away." The altruism required of the program brings as much, if not more, reward to the giver as it does to the receiver. In fact, altruism serves the same reward centers in our brain as the drugs themselves. Altruistic and empathetic socialization is an instinctive quality of ours, and our animal relatives. Altruism and empathetic socialization reduces our stress hormone, cortisol, and increases our comfort hormone, oxytocin, levels. This subject is so provocative and interesting that I have dedicated an entire chapter to its elucidation, Chapter 10.

Attitude of Gratitude

When I have a bad day—and there are plenty, I assure you—and I whine to my sponsor, he will inevitably tell me to "go to my gratitude list," sometimes insisting that I write it down and call him back later in the day. I have found this an invaluable tool for managing my reaction to life and the stress it induces. Gratitude is a frequented Twelve Step oral tradition and reflected in the *Big Book* in the Tenth Step when the authors remark: *"Gratitude for blessings received . . . will be the permanent assets we shall seek."* Twelve steppers will frequently rely on their "attitude of gratitude" when faced with a disappointment or other challenge.

Gratitude is most commonly expressed to the God of one's understanding, but one does not have to have a God to be grateful. The link between spirituality and gratitude has been studied extensively. Gratitude is one of the most common emotions that spiritual practices aim to provoke in worshippers and is regarded as a universal religious sentiment (Emmons, 2005). Studies have found that spirituality is capable of enhancing a person's ability to be grateful; therefore, those who regularly attend spiritual services or engage in spiritual activities are more likely to have a greater sense of gratitude in all areas of life (McCullough, 2002; Emmons, 2000, 2010). Gratitude is viewed as a prized human propensity in the Christian, Buddhist, Muslim, Jewish, and Hindu traditions (Emmons, 2000). The concept of gratitude permeates religious texts, teachings, and traditions with grateful worship to God as the common theme. However, gratitude and God are not inextricable, in as much as "God" and "spirituality" have substantive differences in connotation and expression. Gratitude is an emotional state. I, personally, am grateful to many people, institutions, as well as God. I am grateful to the planet earth for its richness and comfort, a warm sunrise in the morning, etc. Gratitude is an emotional state obtained through spiritual practice.

Gratitude and effects on mental health have been addressed extensively in the psychology literature. The systematic study of gratitude within psychology started only very recently, around the year 2000, as psychology has traditionally been focused more on defining states of pathology and distress rather than focusing on the possible health benefits of positive emotions. At the turn of the century, there was the birth of the "positive psychology movement" which addressed the health benefits of positive affective states, like gratitude (Linley, 2006; Wood, 2007). The study of gratitude within psychology has focused on the understanding of the short-term experience of the emotion of gratitude (state gratitude), individual differences in how frequently people feel gratitude (trait gratitude), and the relationship between these two aspects (Wood, 2008; McCullough, 2004).

Numerous recent studies in the psychology literature have shown that grateful people have higher levels of well-being and that gratitude has one of the strongest links to adaptive, positive mental health of any character trait. Grateful people tend to be happier, less depressed, and less stressed. Grateful people use positive ways of coping with the difficulties they experience in life, being more likely to seek support from other people, reinterpret and grow from the experience, and spend more time focusing on how to deal with a problem, rather than focusing on the problem (Wood, 2007). In this regard, grateful people show less negative coping strategies; that is, they are less likely to try to avoid the problem, deny there is a problem, blame themselves, or use mood-altering substances (Wood, 2007). Those with gratitude express more satisfaction with their lives and social relationships (McCullough, 2002; Wood, 2008; Kashdan, 2006). Grateful individuals expressed better self-acceptance, better control of their environment, personal growth, and purpose in life (Wood, 2007). Grateful people sleep better, because they have less negative thoughts. Negative thoughts incite stress, stimulatory neurotransmitters and hormones, while positive thoughts bring comfort and relaxation (Wood, 2009b).

Two recent studies provide evidence that gratitude may be uniquely important to well-being and satisfaction with life, more so than many other emotions and personality traits. Both studies showed that gratitude was able to explain more well-being and satisfaction with life than the Big Five trait domains (neuroticism, extraversion, openness, agreeableness, and conscientiousness) and thirty of the most commonly studied personality traits (Wood, 2008, 2009a)

Several studies have shown that grateful people are more likely to have higher levels of happiness and lower levels of stress and depression (Seligman, 2005; McCullough, 2004; Wood, 2007). In a recent study by Seligman (2005) of gratitude, participants were randomly assigned to one of six therapeutic intervention conditions designed to improve the participants' overall quality of life. Out of these conditions, it was found that the biggest short-term effects came from a "gratitude visit" where participants wrote and delivered a letter of gratitude to someone in their life. This condition showed a rise in happiness scores and a significant fall in depression scores, results that lasted up to one month after the visit. The longest-lasting effects were caused by the act of writing "gratitude journals" in which participants wrote down three things they were grateful for every day. These participants' happiness scores also increased and continued to increase each time they were tested periodically after the study. In fact, the greatest benefits were usually found to occur around six months after beginning the gratitude journals. Participants were so pleased with the results that, although they were asked to continue the journal for a week, many participants continued to keep the journal long after the study terminated. Similar results have been found from studies conducted by McCullough (2003) and Emmons (2010).

Of particular interest are the multiple studies that have shown gratitude and increased well-being not only for the individual, but for people receiving the gratitude as well (McCullough, 2004, DeSteno, 2010). Gratitude has also been shown to improve a person's altruistic tendencies. One study conducted by DeSteno and Bartlett (2010) found that gratitude is correlated with economic generosity. In this study, using an economic game, increased gratitude was shown to mediate directly increased monetary giving. This study shows that gracious people are more likely to sacrifice individual gains for communal profit. These results show that gracious people are more likely to sacrifice individual gains for communal profit. A study conducted by McCullough, Emmons (2010) found similar correlations between gratitude and empathy, generosity, and helpfulness.

Neither my sponsor nor I had read any of these studies until recently. His advice to me was an oral tradition of Alcoholics Anonymous, which has been around since 1935, and reflective of numerous spiritual practices dating back hundreds, if not thousands of years. My personal lack of gratitude over the years has contributed to substantial personal distress. I am grateful I have found this practice effective in my life today.

"Gratitude is not only the greatest of the
virtues but the parent of all others."
~Cicero, circa 125 BC

"So much has been given to me, I have not time
to ponder over that which has been denied."
~Helen Keller

Chapter 8

Meditation and the Spiritual Experience: Reducing Stress, Finding Serenity, Staying Sober

Step 11 of the Twelve Steps of Alcoholics Anonymous: Sought through prayer and meditation to improve our conscious contact with God, <u>as we understood Him</u>, praying only for knowledge of His will for us and the power to carry that out.

–AA Big Book, p. 59

Carl L.: Chilling Out

Carl L. drank socially for many years. He binged at parties in college and tied it on at holiday parties with his co-workers. He was functional in his car sales job, and at home with his wife and two rambunctious young children. About a year ago, his drinking escalated with the stress of a mortgage and slumping auto sales. He tried AA and "didn't belong there." His family and co-workers noticed his changed appearance and short temper. Months later, they intervened on him and sent him to inpatient treatment. After discharge, he joined AA and found a new group of friends. One of his friends introduced him to a meditation meeting. He loved it so much he went back, again and again. After a few months, Carl learned to meditate on a daily basis and, almost at will when a few moments were free in the workplace or at his busy home. He told me it was the only real way he could relieve his stress. "I do it to chill out," he says, "Without my meditation, I'd be a basket case."

Spiritual Principles and Beliefs

The Eleventh Step of Twelve Step Programs emphasizes continued prayer and meditation as fundamental to maintaining sobriety. Spiritual practices, such as the ability to turn oneself over to a Higher Power or to a God of Our Understanding, are crucial to recovery. In fact, one may say spiritual practices *are* recovery. The authors of the *Big Book* made it clear that this does not mean a single God or religious undertaking. Spiritual beliefs not only embrace the concept of a *power greater than ourselves*, but also encompass a variety of attitudes and perspectives related to developing peace of mind, to interacting empathetically with one's fellows, and to behaving within a moral framework. *Spiritual principles include empathy, honesty, love, tolerance, patience, and acceptance, to name a few. Spiritual practices bring one a sense of peace and wholeness with self and the world. Spiritual practices are comforting; they reduce stress and promote sobriety.*

So how do spiritual beliefs and spiritual practices promote recovery from addiction? Why do they seem to eliminate or mitigate the need for mind-altering and mood-altering drugs or alcohol? These are difficult questions and, certainly, the "right" answer is quite an individual process, based upon beliefs and religious background. This chapter addresses only the biological manifestations of some spiritual experiences. As previously stated, Twelve Step programs do not require belief in God. The authors of the *Big Book* make this clear in the chapter titled "We Agnostics." They could not bear to see an alcoholic robbed of the gift of sobriety because he or she did not believe in God. Although to some (like me) belief in a loving, forgiving God makes the process of recovery easier, agnostics and atheists are welcome in Twelve Step programs and find the same sobriety as the pious.

John F. Kelly (2011), associate professor of psychiatry at Harvard Medical School and the associate director of the Center for Addiction Medicine at Massachusetts General Hospital, showed in a recent study that as attendance of AA meetings increase, so do the participants' spiritual beliefs, especially in those individuals who had low spirituality at the beginning of the study. Kelly said that while spirituality is an important aspect of AA recovery, the organization helps its members in other ways. In his study, the term "spirituality" referred primarily to a belief in a "God of their understanding" and regular prayer and meditation. The researchers assessed more than 1,500 adults throughout their recovery process, with data being gathered at three, six, nine, twelve, and fifteen months. The study utilized data on their attendance to AA meetings, their individual spirituality/religiosity practices, and overall alcohol-use outcomes to determine if spirituality is indeed a mechanism of behavior change. The results showed a strong association between an increase in attendance to AA meetings with increased spirituality, along with a contemporaneous decrease in the frequency and intensity of alcohol use over time.

In this same study, Kelly also reports that AA participation leads to recovery by helping members change their social network and by enhancing individuals' recovery coping skills and motivation for continued abstinence, and by reducing depression and increasing psychological well-being. A most interesting aspect of Dr. Kelly's study was that the same amount of recovery was seen in both agnostics and atheists, which indicates that other AA principles and practices are also important.

Keith Humphreys (2011), a career research scientist with the Veterans Health Administration and professor of psychiatry at Stanford University, has been quoted as saying that *"many people will be surprised that alcoholic patients with little or no interest in spirituality attended AA and seemed to change even more than did those who had a pre-existing, strong sense of spirituality, . . . AA is thus much more broad in its appeal than is commonly recognized."* Dr. Humphreys also noted that while spirituality is an important aspect of recovery, it is still not known how spiritual beliefs work in complement or competition with other recovery methods.

This Doctor's Opinion: Spiritual Practices and Recovery

I believe it is important for the reader to understand, before going further, that I have the highest respect for all spiritual beliefs and religious practices. Our spiritual beliefs and religious affiliations are very personal and of individual importance. Although I was raised Catholic, my beliefs and affiliations have evolved into what I call "Christian lite." I believe in a loving, forgiving God, creator of all things. I believe God has a plan for me, although I have no idea what it encompasses. *I know that if I live a life of integrity, empathy, compassion, and dutiful enterprise, my needs—but maybe not my wants—will be fulfilled.*

My personal quest in recovery, from the perspective of a physician and a scientist, has been to discover the physical, biological correlates of spiritual beliefs and practices. The path of this discovery is *belief neutral,* with findings applicable to those who believe in a single God, multiple gods, or no God at all. The objective of this discovery is to answer two simple questions: How do spiritual practices affect the function of the mind and body? Exactly what physiological and biochemical changes could be occurring with spiritual practices, such as meditation and prayer, that obviate the need for mood-altering substances?

Through my research, I have formulated the opinion that spiritual practices promote recovery in a three-fold manner: First, the practice of meditation, and perhaps some forms of prayer, reduces our mental and physical stress levels, both primarily through changes in cognition and emotional reactivity, and secondarily through reducing cortisol levels and other biological stress responses. Second, some forms of meditation have been shown to stimulate limbic and perilimbic reward centers, releasing dopamine and modulating emotion while strengthening attention and memory. Third, spiritual practices, through improving morals and interpersonal behavior, foster closeness and a sense of community with one's fellows and satisfy our instinctual need for social connection, also reducing stress. (More on this last point in Chapter 9.)

Meditation: Reducing Emotional Distress

The word *"meditation"* is used to describe practices that self-regulate the body and mind, thereby affecting mental events by engaging a specific attentional set. These practices are a subset of those used to induce relaxation or altered states, such as hypnosis, progressive relaxation, and trance-induction techniques. Both basic and clinical research indicate that meditation practices are associated with less emotional distress, more positive states of mind, and better quality of life. In addition, meditation practice can influence the brain, the autonomic nervous system, stress hormones, the immune system, and health behaviors—including eating, sleeping and using substances —in salutary ways. Research on meditation supports the idea that cultivating greater attention, awareness, and acceptance through meditation practice is associated with lower levels of psychological distress, including less anxiety, depression, anger, and worry (Baer, 2003; Brown, 2007; Grossman, 2004). There is rapidly accumulating evidence in the field of complementary health practices that meditation can not only reduce stress and stress-related medical symptoms, but can also enhance positive emotions.

Meditation practices fall into two basic categories: Focused Attention (FA) meditation and Open Monitoring (OM) or Mindful Meditation (MM). Focused Attention (FA) meditation entails voluntary focusing attention on a chosen object or mantra in a sustained fashion. Open Monitoring (OM) meditation involves monitoring the content of experience from moment-to-moment and not reacting to it, either behaviorally or emotionally. One of the goals of the OM technique is to recognize the nature of emotional and cognitive patterns. OM meditation initially involves the use of FA training to calm the mind and reduce distractions, but as FA advances, the cultivation of the monitoring skill per se becomes the main focus of practice. The aim is to reach a state in which no explicit focus on a specific object is retained. One remains only in a passive monitoring state, attentive moment-by-moment to anything that occurs in cognitive experience. These two common styles of meditation are often combined, whether in a single session or over the course of the practitioner's training. These styles are found with some variation in several meditation systems, including the Buddhist Vipassanā and Mahāmudrā, and are also implicated in many popular secular interventions that draw on Buddhist practices. Given the overlap of the FA and OM practices, many authors use the single term *"mindfulness"* to refer to the meditation experience.

"Mindfulness" plays a central role in the teaching of Buddhist meditation where it is affirmed that "correct" or "right" mindfulness is the critical factor in the path to liberation and subsequent enlightenment. The Buddhist term originated from the Pali term *sati* and its Sanskrit variant *sm ti*. The latter was translated into Tibetan as *trenpa* (Wylie: *dran pa*) and Chinese as *nian* These terms best translate into English as "mindfulness." The English term, "mindfulness," has been used for centuries. Described as a calm awareness of one's body functions, feelings, content of consciousness, or consciousness itself, it is the Buddhist tradition's Seventh Element of the Noble Eightfold Path. This is a practice of mindfulness analysis resulting in the development of wisdom (Wynne, 2007).

Mindfulness practice, as inherited from the Eastern Buddhist tradition, is increasingly employed in Western psychology to alleviate a variety of mental and physical conditions. There are a burgeoning number studies that suggest that mindfulness-based approaches are effective in the treatment of obsessive-compulsive disorder (Baer, 2006), anxiety (Hayes,

2004), the prevention of relapse in depression (Segal, 2002; Jain, 7; Segal, 2007) and drug addiction (Marlatt, 1985, 2006).

The common denominator of the benefits of meditation is the reduction of emotional distress. Several studies have been published in this area. One study found that as time in formal meditation practices (body scan, yoga, sitting meditation) increased during an eight-week period, there was increased reported mindfulness and psychological well-being and decreased psychological distress (Carmody, 2008). In a randomized controlled study in students, four weeks of mindfulness meditation, compared with somatic relaxation or a non-intervention control group, reduced emotional distress by decreasing rumination (Jain, 2007). A clinical study of individuals with depression found that eight weeks of mindfulness meditation training significantly reduced ruminative thinking (Ramel, 2004). Rumination has been associated with depression, anxiety and other mood disorders. Mindfulness may also promote better health—in part, by improving sleep quality, which can be disrupted by stress, anxiety and difficulty turning off the mind (Winbush, 2007). Together, these studies indicate that mindfulness meditation reduces obsessive or ruminative thinking and, perhaps most importantly, emotional reactions to these thoughts resulting in reduced emotional distress and improved emotional well-being.

Mindfulness research has found that people who practice mindfulness meditation, irrespective of formal meditation training, report feeling less stressed, anxious and depressed. These same individuals report feeling more joyful, inspired, grateful, hopeful, content, vital, and satisfied with life (Baer, 2006; Brown, 2003; Cardaciotto, 2008; Feldman, 2007; Walach, 2006). In addition to the mental health benefits of dedicated meditation practice, generally requiring a session of thirty minutes or more, simply being in a *mindful state* for brief moments throughout the day is associated with a greater sense of well-being (Lau, 2006).

Research further suggests that people with higher levels of mindfulness are better able to regulate their sense of well-being by virtue of greater emotional awareness, understanding, and acceptance. Individuals report an improved ability to correct or repair unpleasant mood states (Baer, 2008; Brown, 2007; Feldman, 2007). The ability to regulate skillfully one's internal emotional experience in the present moment likely translates into better long-term mental health. Although additional well-designed studies using active control groups are needed to replicate and verify the long-term mental health benefits of mindfulness meditation training, the body of evidence to date supports a relationship between cultivating a more mindful way of being and a tendency to experience less emotional distress, more positive states of mind, and better overall quality of life (Toneatto, 2007).

There are several mindfulness-based training programs—including Mindfulness-Based Stress Reduction (MBSR), Mindfulness-Based Cognitive Therapy (MBCT), Acceptance and Commitment Therapy (ACT), Dialectical Behavior Therapy (DBT), and Mindfulness-Based Eating Awareness Training (MB-EAT)—that have been reported to effectively treat more serious mental health conditions, including anxiety disorders (MBSR; ACT), recurrent major depression (MBCT), chronic pain (MBSR, ACT), borderline personality disorder (DBT), and binge eating disorder (MB-EAT). All employ specific curricula of mindfulness meditation practices, generally individual sessions of approximately thirty minutes, lasting anywhere from ten days to a lifetime (Baer, 2006).

Meditation and the Brain

A number of studies have demonstrated that regular mindfulness meditation training in expert meditators, as well as brief meditation practices in novices, can influence areas of the brain involved in regulating attention, awareness, and emotion (Cahn, 2006; Lutz, 2008a). One key element of mindfulness meditation is the ability to pay attention to the present moment. A recent clinical study found that eight weeks of mindfulness meditation training led to an increased ability to orient one's attention to the present moment, as measured by a laboratory attention test (Jha, 2007). Another experimental study found that compared with a relaxation training control group, five days of integrative meditation training significantly improved the efficiency of executive attention during a computerized attention test (Tang, 2007).

A second key attribute identified in mindfulness meditators is the ability to recognize and accurately label emotions (Analayo, 2003). Brain imaging studies using functional MRI have found that more mindful people appear to have a greater ability to control emotional reactions in the middle part of the brain, namely the amygdala (limbic system) and the dorsal anterior cingulate cortex (the ACC or perilimbic cortex), by engaging the front part of the brain, the prefrontal cortex (PFC), which is associated with attention, concentration, and emotion regulation (Creswell, 2007, 2008). Another study found that employees in a corporate setting showed changes in front brain electrical activity (EEG) following eight weeks of mindfulness meditation training that were consistent with the experience of positive emotions like joy and content (Davidson, 2003).

Over the last decade, Richard Davidson, a psychologist at the University of Wisconsin, Madison, and his colleagues have produced scientific evidence for the theory that meditation produces sustained changes in the brain (Davidson, 2003, 2008, 2010). His research team has hosted scores of Buddhist monks and other meditators for brain scans. The meditation condition was associated with activation in multiple brain regions implicated in monitoring (prefrontal cortex), engaging attention (visual cortex), and attentional orienting (frontal and parietal cortices). Although this meditation-related activation pattern was generally stronger for long-term-practitioners compared with novices, activity in many brain areas involved in FA meditation showed in an inverted U-shaped curve for both classes of subjects. Whereas expert meditators with an average of 19,000 hours of practice showed stronger activation in these areas than the novices, expert meditators with an average of 44,000 practice hours showed less activation. This inverted U-shaped function resembles the learning curve associated with skill acquisition in other domains of expertise, such as language acquisition. The findings support the idea that, after extensive FA meditation training, minimal effort is necessary to sustain attentional focus.

From these scans, he concludes in unpublished postings that strengthening neural systems with the "exercise" of meditation is not fundamentally different from strengthening muscles with physical exercise. Neuroplasticity is a term that is used to describe the brain changes that occur in response to repeated experiences. There are many different mechanisms of neuroplasticity ranging from the growth of new connections to the creation of new neurons. When the framework of neuroplasticity is applied to meditation, neuroscientists agree that the mental training of meditation is fundamentally no different from other forms of skill acquisition that can induce plastic changes in the brain. Indeed, it is the consensus of contemplative neuroscientists that making a habit of meditation can strengthen brain circuits responsible for maintaining concentration, controlling emotions, and generating empathy.

One recent functional MRI study by Davidson's team found that novice meditators stimulated their limbic systems, the brain's emotional network, during the practice of compassion meditation, an ancient Tibetan Buddhist practice. This is no great surprise, given that compassion meditation aims to produce a specific emotional state of intense empathy, sometimes called "loving-kindness." But the study also found that expert meditators, monks with more than 10,000 hours of practice, showed significantly greater activation of their limbic systems than control subjects. The monks appeared to have permanently changed their brains to be more empathetic (Davidson, 2008).

A related study by the same researcher group found that committed meditators experienced sustained changes in baseline brain function, meaning that they had changed the way their brains operated even outside of meditation. These changes included ramped-up activation of a brain region thought to be responsible for generating positive emotions, which they identified as the left frontal lobe. The meditators reported a better state of mind outside of the meditation experience. The researchers found this change in novice meditators who had enrolled in a course in mindfulness meditation that lasted just eight weeks. (Davidson, 2010)

"Effortless concentration" is described in classic meditation texts. In Davidson's laboratory, while the subjects meditated inside the MRI, the researchers periodically blasted them with disturbing noises, such as a baby screaming. Among the experienced meditators, the noise had less effect on the brain areas involved in emotion (the limbic system) and decision-making (frontal cortex) than among novice meditators. Among meditators with more than 40,000 hours of lifetime practice, these areas were hardly affected at all. Most people, if they heard a baby screaming, would have some emotional response and might show activation of the amygdala, the nucleus associated with fear and anger. Davidson found that the highly experienced meditators "hear" the sound, which is reflected in activity in the auditory cortex, but they do not show brain activity in emotional centers in the limbic system. As Davidson notes, any comparison of average middle-aged Americans with people who have meditated daily for decades must try to associate the differences with meditation and not other lifestyle factors, such as isolation or religious faith. Two-thirds of the experienced meditators were Tibetan monks, recruited with the help of the Dalai Lama, and they all had an extremely long history of formal

practice in meditation, as well as substantial lifestyle changes. The lifestyle changes may or may not be the product of their meditation practices.

A third key element of mindfulness meditation is more-refined self-awareness (Kabat-Zinn, 2003). A recent functional MRI study on this topic found that eight weeks of mindfulness meditation training was associated with greater neural activity in two brain regions believed to partially subserve self-awareness, the dorsolateral PFC and the medial PFC, during experiential and narrative self-focus tasks, respectively (Farb, 2007).

A team led by Sara Lazar, Ph.D., a neuroscientist at Massachusetts General Hospital and instructor in psychology at Harvard Medical School, found that meditation increased thickness in the regions of the brain associated with attention and interoception. While previous research with Buddhist monks has demonstrated that long-term meditation may lead to altered brain wave patterns (i.e., EEG's), Dr. Lazar's team hypothesized that long-term meditation practice might also result in changes in the brain's physical structure, possibly reflecting increased use of specific brain regions. Using MRI, Dr. Lazar's group assessed the thickness of the cerebral cortex in twenty participants with extensive experience in mindful meditation. The participants in Dr. Lazar's study were practitioners of Buddhist "insight," or mindful meditation. Two of the study subjects were full-time meditation instructors, two were part-time yoga or meditation teachers, and the remainders were professionals with varied careers. On average, they had nine years of meditation practice, averaging six hours of meditation per week. Unlike Tibetan Buddhist monks, whose lives are devoted to the practice of meditation, practitioners in the United States typically meditate just thirty to forty minutes daily, incorporating the practice into their busy work and family lives (Lazar, 2005)

In this study group the researchers found that brain regions associated with attention, interoception (sensitivity to stimuli originating inside the body), and sensory processing were thicker in the meditation participants than they were in matched controls. These areas included the prefrontal cortex (PFC), which is responsible for planning complex cognitive behaviors, the right anterior insula (INS), which is associated with interoceptive appreciation of bodily sensations and emotions, and the ACC, which is associated with attention. In addition, the researchers found that the differences in cortical thickness were more pronounced in older subjects, suggesting that regular meditation might reduce normal age-related cortical thinning. An independent structural MRI study reported that experienced mindfulness meditators, relative to demographically matched controls, had increased grey matter in brain regions activated in functional MRI experiments during meditation, such as the right anterior insula, and prefrontal cortex (Hölzel, 2007a, 2007b). In unpublished data, this group also found increased grey matter in the hippocampus, associated with memory formation, in long-term meditators.

Researchers are also exploring the individual effects of specific meditation practices on the brain. For example, in experienced meditators, mindful breathing practice, contrasted with mental arithmetic, was associated with increased ACC and dorsomedial PFC activation on functional MRI exams, which may reflect stronger neural suppression of distracting events and emotions, respectively (Hölzel, 2007b). Another functional brain imaging study found that practicing a brief "loving-kindness" meditation activated regions of the brain associated with positive feelings toward others, the ventral striatum (VS) and ACC (Hutcherson, 2008). Loving kindness meditation, traditionally included as part of mindfulness training, is a contemplative practice designed to foster acceptance and compassion for oneself and others (Kabat-Zinn, 1990; Dalai Lama, 2001). Finally, some studies suggest that greater meditation expertise is related to an increased ability to experience shifts in brain activity to the temporal lobe insular cortex and anterior cingulate cortex in response to emotional sounds and associated these findings with compassion (Lutz, 2008b). Other authors, however, have correlated similar findings with attention (e.g., ACC) and emotional regulation (e.g., INS).

Since there is a high concentration of dopaminergic neurons in the ventral striatum (VS), researchers hypothesized the increased neural activity and feelings of well being may be linked to this dopaminergic pathway activation. A study of individuals undergoing guided-attention focused meditation found that dopaminergic changes were associated with the observed increases in VS activity, supporting the hypothesis that endogenous dopamine release may increase during the loss of executive control (from the prefrontal cortex) in meditation (Kjaer et al., 2002). Using, radioactive 11C-raclopride, which selectively and competitively binds to dopamine D2 receptors, researchers showed an approximately 65 percent increase in dopamine release during attention-focused meditation. Increased dopamine release underlying the meditative experience may, therefore, reflect its self-reinforcing nature once proficiency is attained, at least for this form of meditation.

Interesting research has been done using single photon emission computed tomography (SPECT) on Tibetan Buddhist meditators in which participants report "becoming one with" the visualized image (Newberg et al., 2001). (SPECT imaging measures the blood flow in the brain.) The meditators were scanned at baseline and after approximately one hour, when they had indicated entering into the deepest part of their meditation session. Meditation compared with baseline was related to increased blood flow in the ACC, inferior and orbital frontal cortex, dorsolateral prefrontal cortex, midbrain, and thalamus. The midbrain activation may be correlated with alterations in autonomic activity during meditation, namely decreased heart and respiratory rates (Infante, 1998, 2001; Kubota, 2001; Newberg, 2003). Decreased blood flow in the left posterior superior parietal lobe (the precuneus), an area previously shown to correspond with the perception of "self," correlated with the blood flow increase observed in the left dorsolateral prefrontal cortex. *It is tempting to conjecture that these results apparently show the neural correlate of the popular Twelve-Step slogan, "getting out of self," reinforced to recovering addicts and alcoholics by their sponsors as a philosophy of reducing selfishness and promoting selflessness.*

Researchers have also studied practitioners of a form of Kundalini yoga, entailing a "mantra-guided" meditation combined with heightened breath awareness, with functional MRI (Lazar et al., 2000). The control activity was the mental construction of animal names. Each of the five meditation participants had practiced Kundalini yoga for at least four years. The scan findings during meditation, compared with control conditions, produced activity increases in the putamen, midbrain, anterior cingulate cortex, hippocampal and parahippocampal areas, as well as areas within the prefrontal and parietal cortices. Assessment of early versus late meditation states found robust activity increases in these areas, a greater number of activation foci, larger signal changes, and higher proportion of individuals with significant changes during the late meditation states. These results suggest that, with increased meditation time, individuals produce altered brain states that may index changed states of consciousness as they continue their meditation. Indeed, the major increased activity areas were those subserving attention (frontal and parietal cortices, particularly the dorsolateral PFC) and those subserving arousal and autonomic control (limbic regions, midbrain, and ACC).

Other studies have been conducted on individuals with extensive training in Kundalini (mantra-based) or Vipassana (mindfulness-based) meditation. The meditators were imaged with functional MRI during meditation and several control tasks (e.g., simple rest, generation of a random list of numbers, and paced breathing (Lazar, 2003). The results indicated that each style of meditation was associated with a different pattern of brain activity. In the two meditator groups, similar but non-overlapping frontal and parietal cortices as well as subcortical structures were engaged, and these patterns differed from those observed during control tasks. The main area of common activation was the dorsal anterior cingulate cortex. Vipassana participants experienced little or no decrease in respiratory rate, whereas Kundalini participants typically had decreases of greater than four breaths per minute during meditation compared with baseline.

There are a handful of functional MRI studies on Zen meditation practitioners. As the name "Zen" implies, sitting meditation is a core aspect of Zen practice. In Japanese, this is called *zazen*, and in Chinese, it is called *zuòchán* (坐禅), both simply meaning "sitting dhyāna." During this sitting meditation, practitioners usually assume a position such as the lotus, half-lotus, Burmese, or seiza postures. To regulate the mind, awareness is directed toward counting, attending to the breath, or focusing one's energy center below the navel. In one study, Zen practitioners were assessed with functional MRI using an on–off design of forty five second blocks in which meditators counted their breath as in normal practice during three meditation periods and engaged in random thoughts during the intervening three forty five second rest periods. Compared with the resting state, meditation showed increased activity in the dorsolateral prefrontal cortex and ventral striatum (VS). Decreased activity was found in the right anterior superior occipital gyrus (visual cortex) and anterior cingulate cortex (Ritskes, 2003). Activity decrease in the anterior cingulate cortex was not as strong as the increase in the dorsolateral PFC. The authors of this study attributed the ACC decrease to a decrease in the experience of "will" in the meditative state. Given the evidence for increased ACC activation in other studies, this finding may have been related to the very short periods of time allotted for the successive Zen states.

Another functional MRI study was conducted on five Zen mindfulness meditation practitioners. In this study, two repetitions of the onset of meditation were assessed as successive forty-five-second on-off stages of meditation (Baerentsen, 2001). Activations were found in the paired hippocampi, left frontal, right temporal, and ACC, with deactivations in the visual cortex. The significant increased activations in ACC and prefrontal and orbitofrontal cortex have been found in the majority of non-guided meditation studies (Herzog et al., 1990; Khushu, 2000; Lazar, 2000, 2003).

Besides the importance of ACC activation as a marker of the increased attentional focus in meditative states, this structure also appears related to feelings of love and positive affection, likely due to the attentional demands of these emotions (Bartels, 2000, 2004). Some meditators consistently report such feelings during meditation (Mahesh, 1963), although these experiences are not the explicit goal in the most commonly practiced meditation techniques, such as Transcendental, Vipassana, and Zen (Goleman, 1996; Wallace, 1999).

Prefrontal cortical areas are activated in attention-focusing tasks likely due to the effortful intentional activity involved in most meditative practices (Frith, 1991; Pardo, 1991). Studies comparing internally generated versus externally generated word rehearsal demonstrated a shift from medial prefrontal activation to more lateral areas (Crosson, 2001). The increased activity of the dorsolateral prefrontal cortex may contribute to the self-regulation of brain functioning, because it has been shown to contribute to self-regulating emotional reactions (Beauregard, 2001; Levesque, 2003), and decreased emotional reactivity is reported to ensue from meditative practice (Goleman, 2003; Wallace, 2000).

Functional MR activity in the posterior superior parietal lobe (responsible for spatial processing) during visual-spatial orientation tasks has been observed to decrease in conjunction with the increase in left dorsolateral prefrontal cortex, suggesting a neural basis for the altered sense of spatial awareness present in the meditative state (Cohen, 1996; D'Esposito, 1998). Several investigations have reported decreased posterior superior parietal lobe activity associated with decreased experience of self-non-self boundaries (d'Aquili, 1993, 1998, 2000).

Overall, it appears that focused, concentrative/attentive meditation practices can increase one's ability to maintain steady attention on a chosen object, like the breath or another person, whereas open awareness meditation or mindfulness practices can increase one's ability to flexibly monitor and redirect attention when it becomes distracted, particularly by internally generated emotions (Lutz, 2008a). Based on the function and structural MRI findings presented above, not only is it possible to train the mind to change the brain, but, in fact, one's ability to do so may get stronger as one gains meditation experience. Areas consistently "strengthened" include the prefrontal cortex, which is responsible for planning complex cognitive behaviors, and the temporal lobe insula, which is associated with interoceptive appreciation of bodily sensations and emotions and the frontal lobe anterior cingulate cortex, which is associated with attention.

Brain Regions Affected by Meditation

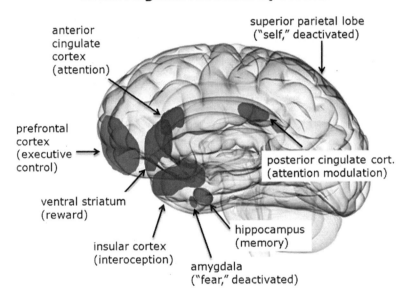

anterior cingulate cortex (attention)

superior parietal lobe ("self," deactivated)

prefrontal cortex (executive control)

posterior cingulate cort. (attention modulation)

ventral striatum (reward)

insular cortex (interoception)

hippocampus (memory)

amygdala ("fear," deactivated)

Effect of Prayer on the Brain

A limited number of medical imaging studies have been carried out with Christian prayer practices. In one study, functional MRI exams performed on religious individuals were compared with a nonreligious group during recitation versus reading of Psalm 23, a popular German nursery rhyme, and a telephone book (Azari, 2001). The religious individuals reported achieving a "religious state" while reciting Psalm 23, and significant activations were found in the dorsolateral and dorsomedial prefrontal cortex, and right medial parietal lobe compared with other readings and with nonreligious control individuals. The increases in PFC were especially strong and significantly increased relative to all comparisons. In contrast, the non-religious individuals reported experiencing a happy state in reciting the nursery rhyme, which was associated with PFC, parietal and amygdala activation that, in turn, the authors correlated with a positive affective state.

In another study, Franciscan nuns praying were assessed with SPECT blood-flow imaging in a fashion similar to Tibetan Buddhist meditators (Newberg, 2003b). They engaged in centering prayer, which "requires focused attention on a phrase from the Bible" and involves "opening themselves to being in the presence of God" and "loss of the usual sense of space," making it a relatively good approximation of some forms of mantra-based meditational practices. Compared with baseline, scans during prayer demonstrated increased blood flow in the PFC, inferior parietal lobes, and inferior frontal lobes, although decreased flow in the superior parietal lobe. There was a strong correlation between increased blood flow in the PFC and decreased blood flow in the superior parietal lobe (spatial awareness, "self").

The findings of these and other studies of prayer bear some similarity to studies in meditators, although they cannot be directly compared with them, as prayer involves recursive thought whereas meditation does not. The findings in prayer further suggest that meditative/spiritual experiences are partly mediated through a deactivation of the superior parietal lobe, which normally helps to generate the normal sense of spatial awareness and "self" (d'Aquili, 2000).

It is my personal belief that prayer, in and of itself, does not cause things to change in the world, but rather prayer causes things to change within ourselves which, in turn, change our behaviors, the way people respond to us, the way we perform our duties, etc. Then, and only then, do things in the world change. The founders of AA also appear to share this philosophy, as they state in the Twelve Steps and Twelve Traditions: *"So we of AA do obey spiritual principles, first because we must, and ultimately because we love the kind of life such obedience brings"* (p. 174). Bill W. and Dr. Bob, AA's founding fathers, go on to state that we alcoholics cannot pray solely for our alcoholism to miraculously vanish. In the *Big Book*, they state, *"I've prayed to God on hangover mornings and sworn that I'd never touch another drop, but by nine o'clock I'd be boiled as an owl."* (*AA Big Book*, p. 158) Nonetheless, the founders of AA fully recognized the strength of prayer and meditation in recovery and thus promoted their use in the Eleventh Step.

Louis Teresi, MD

Meditation and the Body: Reducing Stress

There is vast wealth of scientific evidence to support the therapeutic effect of mindfulness meditation on stress-related medical conditions, including psoriasis (Kabat-Zinn, 1998), type 2 diabetes (Rosenzweig, 2007), fibromyalgia (Grossman, 2007), rheumatoid arthritis (Pradhan, 2007; Zautra, 2008), chronic low back pain (Morone, 2008), and attention-deficit hyperactivity disorder (Zylowska et al., 2008). Traditionally, meditative techniques have been taught and practiced through formal and in-formal meditation centers. More recently, meditation has also become a component of many therapeutic programs; in 1997, over 240 meditation programs were a part of U.S. health care systems, and the basics of meditation are taught in many U.S. medical schools. In addition, research has consistently shown that mindfulness training reduces symptoms of stress and negative mood states, and increases emotional well-being and quality of life, among persons with chronic illness (Brown, 2007; Grossman, 2004; Ludwig, 2008; Shigaki, 2006). The use of mindfulness training in treating specific pain conditions, hypertension, myocardial ischemia, weight control, irritable bowel syndrome, insomnia, human immunodeficiency virus (HIV), and substance abuse is presently under investigation in research supported by the National Institutes of Health (Ludwig, 2008).

The beneficial physical effects of meditation may occur, in part, by learning how to cope better with the inevitable stresses of daily life, which take their toll in deteriorated quality of life (lack of sleep, reduced work productivity, reduced sex drive), increased cardiovascular disease, compromised immune system, and of course, increased incidence of substance abuse. Theoretical psychological models of meditation have endeavored to explain empirical observations of its positive effects by articulating the role of improved cognitive skills, like "decentering" (Teasdale, 2002) or "reperceiving" (Shapiro, 2006), and adaptive coping processes, like "positive reappraisal" (Garland, 2007). It has been postulated that meditation may preempt stress-related illness through psychological, biological and behavioral pathways, including: (1) clarifying primary appraisal of precipitating stressors, (2) facilitating accurate secondary appraisal of stressor demands and coping resources, (3) mitigating dysfunctional coping styles (i.e. catastrophizing and ruminating), and (4) enhancing adaptive coping processes, such as positive reappraisal. The objective of these psychological adaptations is reducing stress and its psychological and physiological activation (Garland, 2007).

Laboratory research is beginning to reveal some of the biological pathways through which mindfulness training may have a positive impact on physical health and healing processes. For example, an eight-week mindfulness meditation training study by Davidson and colleagues (2003) showed that individuals who had the largest shifts in frontal brain activity also had the strongest antibody responses to a flu vaccine. That study was the first to show that mindfulness meditation can change the immune system in a way that might bolster resistance to disease. Research on patients with HIV infection further indicates that mindfulness meditation training may produce beneficial effects on the immune system, including increased natural killer cell activity, an important first line of defense against viral infection, as well as increased production of β-chemokines, molecules that block HIV from infecting healthy immune cells (Robinson, 2003). A different study on adults with HIV infection suggested that mindfulness meditation training may protect against the loss of "helper" T-cells over time, a primary measure of HIV disease progression (Creswell, 2009). Another study found that adults who reported home practice times above the median during a six-week compassion meditation training program exhibited significantly lower stress-induced levels of negative emotion and inflammation (interleukin-6) compared to controls (Pace et al., 2008). More recent mindfulness meditation training studies in people with serious medical conditions—including breast cancer, prostate cancer, and other types of cancer—have documented lower levels of cortisol, the primary stress hormone, and normalized immune function, measured by natural killer cell activity and pro-inflammatory cytokine levels (Carlson, 2007; Witnek-Janusek, 2008).

Other research studies have shown that mindfulness meditation can alter autonomic and neuroendocrine system functioning, both at rest and when stressed. For example, one study found that mindful meditation produced greater increases in parasympathetic nervous system activity, as reflected in decreased heart rate and blood pressure, than a progressive muscle relaxation technique (Ditto, 2006). Another study showed that five days of meditation training, including mindfulness, significantly reduced the cortisol response to acute mental stress relative to a relaxation training control group that did not receive mindfulness or meditation instruction (Tang, 2007). *Taken together, these experimental studies indicate that mindfulness practices may promote health, in part, by attenuating stress reactivity and stimulating parasympathetic tone, perhaps more strongly than relaxation techniques.*

In the largest and most widely quoted of the studies of the effects of mindful meditation on physiological stress parameters, Dr. Sudsuang (Department of Physiology and Anatomy, Faculty of Medicine, Chulalongkorn University, Bangkok, Thailand) studied fifty-two males twenty to twenty-five years of age practicing Dhammakaya Buddhist meditation, and thirty males of the same age group not practicing meditation as a control group (Sudsuang, 1991). All practitioners had at least five years of mindful meditation experience, and most meditated on a daily basis. These researchers found that after meditation, serum cortisol levels were significantly reduced, serum total protein level significantly increased, and systolic pressure, diastolic pressure, and pulse rate significantly reduced. Measures of respiratory function, including vital capacity, tidal volume, and maximal voluntary ventilation, were significantly lower after meditation than before, consistent with relaxation and reduced stress. There were also significant decreases in reaction time after meditation practice, indicative of lowered sympathetic tone. *Results from these studies indicate that practicing Dhammakaya Buddhist meditation produces biochemical and physiological changes consistent with reduced physiological stress.*

A research group from the Department of Psychology at the University of Westminster, in an investigation designed to explore the impact of a five-week kinesthetic meditation training program, studied fifty-seven healthy undergraduate students, allocated to either a control group (n = 26) or meditation group (n = 31) (Bullen, 2006). Salivary cortisol, stress and arousal were measured before and after the five weeks, during which the participants could attend kinesthetic meditation training sessions for one hour each week, as well as practice at home with the aid of a CD. There were no statistically significant differences between the groups in demographics or any of the measures at the start of the investigation. Cortisol secretion in the meditation group was lower on the day of the final kinesthetic meditation session compared with on a typical day in the same week and the control group measured in the same week. The authors concluded that the benefit derived from kinesthetic meditation sessions was clearly measurable on the day of the session, but not detectable on a day when participants were not exposed to the program. The data suggests brief periods of kinesthetic meditation training over a short period of time can improve objective measures of stress.

Meditation for "Breaking" Habitual Behaviors

A fundamental principle of meditation, particularly mindfulness meditation, is the cultivation of "non-reactivity" or equanimity to intrusive thoughts. Specifically, mindfulness meditation teaches one to pay attention to and acknowledge both one's inner experience and the outer world, without necessarily reacting. The ability to simply observe and accurately sense thoughts, emotions, and physical sensations, without having to change them, or *act* on them, can be instrumental in breaking habitual behavior patterns. Too many people smoke a cigarette when feeling stressed, eat comfort food when feeling sad or lonely, or turn to alcohol or other substances to "numb out" when feeling overwhelmed.

Behavioral research has suggested that mindfulness training may help people to experience stress and negative emotions without acting impulsively and self-destructively in their attempt to self-sooth (Brown, 2007). For example, some of the studies to date have found that people trained in mindfulness show a better ability to quit smoking (Davis, 2007), decrease binge eating (Kristeller, 2006), and reduce alcohol and illicit substance use (Bowen, 2006). At least one study has shown that reduced substance use following mindfulness training was partially explained by acceptance, rather than avoidance, of unwanted thoughts (Bowen, 2007).

Mindfulness-Based-Stress-Reduction Therapy for Sobriety

The theoretical framework for mindfulness meditation suggests that it may be a promising approach to treating addictive disorders (Breslin, 2002; Marlatt, 2007). The "observe and accept" approach, a characteristic of meditation, refers to being fully present and attentive to current experience but not being pre-occupied by it. Meditation is often contrasted with everyday, habitual, mental functioning or being on "auto-pilot." As such, meditation may be a valuable technique for addicted individuals, whose condition is often associated with unwanted thoughts, emotions and sensations (e.g., craving), and the tendency to be on "auto-pilot" with a pre-occupation for the "next fix," rather than "being in the present moment."

Mindfulness-Based Stress Reduction (MBSR) has been the most widely studied meditation method employed in substance use disorders (SUD's).

MBSR has been shown to be effective or potentially effective for many mental health and medical conditions (Kabat-Zinn, 1990) Originally developed for management of chronic pain and stress-related disorders, MBSR is the most frequently cited method of meditation training in the medical context (Baer, 2006) and has a published curriculum (Kabat-Zinn, 1990). The usual MBSR course consists of eight weekly, therapist-led group sessions (2 to 2.5 hours per session), one full-day retreat (7 to 8 hours) and daily home assignments.

Dr. Aleksandra Zgierska of the University of Wisconsin School of Medicine recently performed an exhaustive meta-analysis of the effectiveness of MBSR in SUDs (Zgierska, 2009). To date, seven randomized clinical trials have been done evaluating the MBSR program for SUDs. Overall, these studies included a total of 383 adult subjects (63 percent female), followed for an average of thirty-eight weeks after initial entry—from eight (Avants, 2005; Margolin, 2006) to sixty-eight (Linehan, 2002, 1999) weeks—offering the most detailed assessment of MBSR treatments. Six studies evaluated severely impaired populations, and one (N = 38) focused on tobacco-dependent adults. Six of seven studies used a two-arm approach (comparing two treatment groups), and one used a three-arm design (comparing three groups) (Hayes, 2004). Three studies compared MBSR plus "standard of care" (SOC) with SOC alone (Alterman, 2004; Margolin, 2006), with both MBSR and SOC provided at the same clinical site. SOC practices included group as well as individual therapy in a cognitive-behavioral therapy format. One study compared MBSR with SOC, with SOC subjects referred out for therapy as a control population (Linehen, 1999). Finally, four studies (Avants, 2005; Gifford, 2004; Hayes, 2004; Linehan, 1999) compared MBSR with an active intervention: three to a different therapy (behavioral (Hayes, 2004; Linehan, 1999) or pharmacotherapy (Gifford, 2004)), and one compared MBSR delivered in "individual" versus "individual plus group format" therapies (Avants, 2005).

All studies reported some positive results for the MBSR-treated groups. Compared with SOC treatments, the MBSR treatments showed positive effects as reflected in abstinence rates in the follow-up period after completion of therapy. Differential improvement in both substance use-related and other outcomes was noted in five of seven studies (Gifford, 2004; Hayes, 2004; Linehan, 1999, 2002; Margolin 2006). One study (Alterman, 2004) noted a differential improvement in medical symptom severity only, and one study (Avants, 2005), comparing MBSR therapy with "individual" therapy to "individual plus group" therapy did not find differences between the study groups, but noted pre-post improvements in substance-use outcomes for all treatment groups.

Overall, randomized clinical trials using SOC (i.e., cognitive-behavioral therapies) (Gifford, 2004; Hayes, 2004; Linehan, 1999; Margoli,n 2006) as a comparison group tended to report greater statistically significant sobriety rates for the MBSR-treated groups. A study by Hayes et al. (2004), with the largest sample size of 124 poly-substance-abusing methadone-maintenance patients, suggested that MBSR plus SOC may result in a substantial reduction of substance use compared with SOC alone. The reported difference in sobriety rates was 33 percent greater in the MBSR plus SOC group compared with the SOC group; that is, 33 percent more patients remained sober in the follow-up period with MBSR. This finding was consistent across three other randomized clinical trials comparing MBSR with SOC (30 percent) (Linehan, 1999; Margolin, 2006), or with pharmacotherapy with medical management (12 to 20 percent) (Gifford, 2004). Regarding non-substance-use–related measures, MBSR subjects increased their motivation for HIV prevention, their spiritual practices, and showed a cognitive shift from "addict" to "spiritual qualities" compared with SOC subjects (Margolin, 2006). They also significantly improved their psychological adjustment to life stresses as measured by the global adjustment and global social adjustment scale scores (Linehan, 1999).

Dr. Aleksandra Zgierska also analyzed four controlled nonrandomized trials described by six articles (Altner, 2002; Bowen, 2006, 2007; Marcus, 2001; Margolin, 2007; Simpson, 2007), four case series described by six articles (Bootzin, 2005; Davis, 2007; Marcus, 2003; Stevens, 2007; Zgierska, 2008; Haynes, 2006), and one case report (Twohig, 2007) of the efficacy of MBSR in SUDs. These studies included 609 subjects, 13 to 67 years old, suffering from various SUDs, and recruited from the outpatient treatment (Marcus, 2001, 2003; Margolin, 2007; Bootain, 2005; Stevens, 2007; Zgierska, 2008; Haynes, 2006), community (Altner, 2002; Davis, 2007), or jail (Simpson, 2007; Bowen, 2006) settings. Collectively they reported overall positive outcomes for MBSR methods. On average, substance use tended to decrease at follow-up compared with baseline (Altner, 2002; Zgierska, 2008; Davis, 2007) or compared with a control group by 47 to 56 percent in short follow-up periods of 60 to 112 days. Severity of potential relapse triggers (such as stress, mental health and sleep problems, and certain coping styles) also tended to improve compared with both baseline and control conditions in all studies.

In Zgierska's 2008 study of MBSR in alcoholics, participants reported they were abstinent on 94.5 percent of study days, with 47 percent reporting complete abstinence and 47 percent reporting one or more heavy drinking days. Their severity of depression, anxiety, stress, and craving (documented relapse triggers) decreased, and the degree of mindfulness increased. The meditation course was rated as a very important and useful relapse-prevention tool; participants reported being very likely to continue meditating. Gaining skills to reduce stress, coping with craving, and good group support were the most common qualitative comments about the course value. Zgierska compared "relapsers" (subjects reporting at least one heavy drinking day during the study) with non-relapsers and found that relapsers had more severe symptoms of anxiety, depression, and craving, reported lower degree of mindfulness, and meditated fewer minutes per day. The authors also reported that drinking level as well as the change in drinking correlated to the severity of relapse risk factors, such as anxiety, depression, stress, and craving and the change in their severity, respectively. In turn, severity of relapse risk factors increased as the intensity of a daily meditation practice decreased. Compared with baseline, at sixteen weeks, interleukin-6 levels decreased; cortisol levels were reduced but not significantly. In another uncontrolled study of MBSR intervention, SUD-affected residents of a therapeutic community showed a decrease in an awakening salivary cortisol level compared with baseline (Marcus, 2003).

Sarah Bowen and colleagues (2006), of the University of Washington, Department of Psychology evaluated the effectiveness of a ten-day mindfulness meditation course on substance use and psychosocial outcomes in a jail population, followed for a fifteen-month period. Results indicate that after release from jail, participants in the mindful meditation course, as compared with those in a treatment-as-usual control condition, showed significant reductions in alcohol, marijuana, and crack cocaine use in four of five outcome measures. Mindfulness meditation participants showed decreases in alcohol-related problems and psychiatric symptoms as well as increases in positive psychosocial outcomes.

In a later study, Dr. Bowen suggested that the advantage of mindfulness meditation was its emphasis on acceptance on, rather than suppression of, unwanted thoughts (Bowen, 2007). Her research group noted that previous studies have demonstrated that attempts to suppress thoughts about using substances may actually lead to increases in substance use (Wegner, 1987, 1997). Her 2007 study showed significant decreases in active avoidance of thoughts in subjects participating in a ten-day mindfulness meditation course when compared with controls. Mindfulness meditation course participants did not report a significant decrease in intrusive thoughts, only their reaction to them. Thus, the frequency of unwanted thoughts may not be as important as the manner in which an individual copes with those thoughts. The process of passively accepting rather than actively suppressing unwanted thoughts likely partially accounted for the relationship between participation in the meditation course and reduced alcohol use and consequences three months following release from jail.

Bowen's results provide support for the hypothesis that active thought avoidance or suppression may be an important component in the relationship between the persistent mental obsession to drink and actual alcohol use (Witkiewitz, 2005) and that this obsession may be mitigated through mindfulness meditation. Only one uncontrolled trial of alcoholics treated with MBSR therapy, adjunctive to SOC, assessed craving severity and the degree of mindfulness (Zgierska, 2008). Although craving severity decreased, this change was not statistically significant. The degree of mindfulness, or the ability to be attentive to a present-moment experience in daily life, improved, and this change correlated with improved stress management at sixteen-week follow-up (Zgierska, 2008).

Although long-term MBSR practice patterns have not been assessed in the context of SUDs, its use in other clinical samples suggests that MBSR can have long-lasting effects. For example, after a meditation course, 60 to 90 percent of subjects still meditated up to four years later, and reported that the course "had lasting value" and was highly important (Baer, 2003). Patient satisfaction is an important consideration when choosing between treatment alternatives (Kadzin, 1994). MBSR also appears safe. Rigorous studies have not reported any side effects or adverse events.

The theoretical framework of mindfulness meditation behind MBSR, as well as early studies, supports the use of MBSR for SUD's and suggests unique therapeutic properties of MBSR. MBSR stands out as distinctive and, in many ways, different from other existing behavioral modalities, specifically from cognitive behavioral therapy (CBT) that is commonly used to treat SUD's. While CBT promotes adaptive, antecedent-focused coping strategies (e.g., targeting emotion cues), mindfulness meditation targets maladaptive, response-focused strategies, such as emotional avoidance, impulse control, and reduction of emotional and physiological stress. Virtually all studies to date support MBSR in an integrated approach to SUD's. MBSR improves overall treatment efficacy by increasing awareness of sensations, such as craving, emotional states, and reducing emotional and physiological stress.

The latest scientific research on mindfulness meditation has demonstrated beneficial effects on several aspects of whole-person health, including the mind, the brain, the body, and behavior. Clinical trials and laboratory studies alike suggest that the mechanisms of mindfulness involve not only relaxation and stress reduction, but important shifts in cognition, emotion, biology, and behavior that may work synergistically to improve health and maintain sobriety. There is also emerging evidence that mindfulness meditation is associated with greater meaning and peace in one's life (spirituality), as well as enhanced relationships with others (Carmody, 2008; Carson, 2004).

Chapter 9

Instinctive Empathetic Socialization: The Science of Trust, Empathy and Altruism; Why Twelve-Step Groups Work

"Meeting makers make it."   *"Pain shared is pain halved."*
~Old AA adages

Joe M.: Almost "Going Out"

Joe M. is a fiftyish man, married for fifteen years to the same wife, and has three healthy children. He owns a small business in Southern California, which he has run successfully since its inception. An alcoholic who reached his bottom in a jail cell for a DUI, Joe joined AA, got a sponsor, worked the steps, went to meetings, and is now ten years sober. About four years ago, Joe and another AA member got in a mild argument at Joe's favorite meeting. Joe decided to "vote with his feet" and left the meeting. He knew he had to 'work-through' the resentment, which he did with his sponsor. He let it go. Joe decided to lighten up on his meeting schedule and he went without regular meetings for almost two years. Over that time he continued to work the steps with his sponsor, prayed and meditated, but attended only scattered AA meetings. He didn't drink, but he felt his comfort and serenity level slowly erode over that time and, on many occasions, was very close to taking a drink. He tells me he had a persistent sense of distress and his coping skills were waning. He "re-committed" to his original group, became friends with the fellow AA member involved in the former conflict, and regained his serenity, his "emotional sobriety." Two years later, Joe remains a content,

235

sober member of AA. Joe told me *"Meetings make me feel good . . . I feel comfortable here."*

Groups and Recovery

Joe's experience is typical in the recovering community. *It is common for a participant in Twelve-Step groups to say that participating in the groups makes them "feel good," and they "get centered" from the group, but they cannot articulate why this is so.* It is also not uncommon for participants to have affectionate attachment to the group as whole and its individual members. Group members are known give each other gentle hugs of affection and the words "I love you guys," or similar, are used liberally, in a non-romantic context, of course. (Romantic attachments are strongly discouraged in Twelve Step recovery groups.)

The natural propensity of human beings to congregate makes group therapy and self-help groups, like Twelve Step groups, a powerful therapeutic tool for treating substance abuse, one that is well-recognized to be as or more successful than individual therapy. One reason for this efficacy is that groups intrinsically have many rewarding benefits. Our need for human contact is biologically determined; we are, from the start, social creatures. Socialization instincts are a requirement for survival in all mammalian populations. Belonging to a group facilitates foraging for food, protection from predators, reproduction, and caring for the young. Isolation in mammals and humans results in increased physiological stress, which has deleterious health consequences and can be deadly. In fact, the higher along the phylogenetic tree we look, the more advanced and complex socialization skills become. *Humans must be social to survive.*

Human beings' innate drive to socialize and propensity to congregate has proven to be a powerful therapeutic tool. The lives of individuals are shaped, for better or worse, by their experiences in groups. People are born into groups. Throughout life, we join groups. Our lives are profoundly influenced by family, religious, social, and cultural groups that constantly shape behavior, self-image, and both physical and mental health. Groups can support individual members in times of pain and trouble, and they can help people grow in ways that are healthy and creative.

Self-help groups and facilitated formal therapy groups can be a compelling source of persuasion, stabilization, and support. Groups organized around therapeutic goals can enrich members with insight and guidance; and during times of crisis, groups can comfort and guide people who otherwise might be unhappy or lost. The potential curative forces inherent in a group can be harnessed and directed to foster healthy attachments, provide positive peer reinforcement, act as a forum for self-expression, and teach new social skills. In short, group therapy or self-help groups can provide a wide range of therapeutic services, comparable in efficacy to those delivered in individual therapy. They reduce isolation and enable members to witness the recovery of others, and these qualities draw members into a culture of recovery. Groups offer support, gratification, and identification. This capacity of groups to bond individuals to shared therapeutic goals is an important asset in recovery.

Group therapy and addiction treatment are natural allies. One reason is that people who abuse substances often are more likely to remain abstinent and committed to recovery when treatment is provided in groups, apparently because of rewarding and therapeutic forces associated with affiliation. The effectiveness of group therapy in the treatment of substance abuse also can be attributed to the nature of addiction and several factors associated with it, including (but not limited to) depression, anxiety, isolation, denial, shame, temporary cognitive impairment, and character pathology (personality disorder, structural deficits, or an unhealthy sense of self). Whether a person abuses substances or not, these problems often respond better to group treatment than to individual therapy (Kanas, 1982; Kanas, 1983, Scheidlinger 2000; Toseland, 1986).

There is a wide variety of groups available to the addict and alcoholic: Self-help groups are the most popular and available, represented by Twelve-Step Groups, such as AA, NA, etc. *Over 200 self-help organizations, often known as fellowships, with a worldwide membership of millions, now employ Twelve-Step principles for recovery.* Professionally-facilitated groups available through licensed professionals include: psycho-educational groups, which teach about substance abuse; skills development groups, which hone the skills necessary to break free of addictions; cognitive–behavioral groups, which rearrange patterns of thinking and action that lead to addiction; and interpersonal process groups which enable clients to discuss relational and other life problems. All groups can be therapeutic, as long as there is a common therapeutic objective, such as sobriety. It is universally agreed amongst addiction specialists that for a group to be effective there *must be some emotional attachment* to other group members, a group leader, or the group as a whole. This emotional attachment should be at the level of empathy, but not exclusive of compassion.

Treatment professionals have described numerous advantages to using groups in substance abuse treatment: (Brown, 1977; Flores, 1997; Vannicelli, 1992):

- *Groups provide positive peer support and pressure to abstain from substances of abuse.* The addict or alcoholic is known to suffer from denial and poor-decision making abilities. Groups help break down this denial and offer rational solutions to problems.
- *Groups can effectively confront individual members about substance abuse and other harmful behaviors.*
- *Groups reduce the sense of isolation that most people who have substance abuse disorders experience.*
- *Groups enable people who abuse substances to witness the recovery of others.*
- *Groups help members learn to cope with their substance abuse and other problems by allowing them to see how others deal with similar problems.*
- *Groups can provide useful information to addicts who are new to recovery.*
- *Groups provide feedback concerning the values and abilities of other group members.* This information helps members improve their conceptions of self or modify faulty, distorted conceptions. In terms of process groups in particular, as specific themes emerge in a member's group experience, repetitive feedback from multiple group members can chip away at those faulty or distorted conceptions in slightly different ways until they not only are correctable, but also the very process of correction and change is revealed through the examination of the group processes.
- *Groups offer family-like experiences.* Groups can provide the support and nurturance that may have been lacking in group members' families of origin. The group also gives members the opportunity to practice healthy ways of interacting with their families.
- *Groups encourage, coach, support, and reinforce as members undertake difficult or anxiety-provoking tasks.*
- *Groups offer members the opportunity to learn or relearn the social skills they need to cope with everyday life instead of resorting to substance abuse.* Group members can learn by observing others,

being coached by others, and practicing skills in a safe and supportive environment.

- *Groups can add needed structure and discipline to the lives of people with substance use disorders, who often enter treatment with their lives in chaos.*

- *Groups instill hope, a sense that "If he can make it, so can I."* Process groups can expand this hope to dealing with the full range of what people encounter in life, overcome, or cope with.

- *Groups often support and provide encouragement to one another outside the group setting.* For interpersonal process groups, though, outside contacts may or may not be disallowed, depending on the particular group contract or agreements.

Without the group's empathy, stated or implied, none of the aforementioned bullet points can be achieved. As we will explore in this chapter, it is the opinion of this author that the foundation for the effectiveness of Twelve Step and other recovery groups is *"empathic socialization."* Being present in a group empathetic to one's emotional pain, one's distress, provides a natural and healthy alternative to substances of abuse. In the text that follows, we will explore a large body of scientific observation and research in support of the following thesis:

Positive socializing experiences received in support and therapeutic groups, such as praise, affection and empathic understanding, activate the brain's reward centers as much as other natural rewards and similar to addictive substances. More importantly, belonging to an empathetic group reduces stress, a predominant cause and catalyst of addiction. Positive, empathetic socialization experiences have been shown to have a powerful antistress effect through reduction of CRF and cortisol and activation of other hormones, like oxytocin, which have an anxiolytic effect, producing feelings of comfort and calm. *Thus, the rewarding and stress-reducing characteristics of group affiliation mitigate the desire for mood-altering substances and promote emotional recovery.*

I would like to emphasize that an individual participant in any group must have the perception of *empathy from the group* for the rewarding and antistress effects to be obtained. For this reason, the group members must share a common purpose; i.e. recovery from substance dependence, and usually sobriety from a particular addictive substance, group of substances, or behavior. An individual with substance dependence receives little from sharing their distress with a group that has no substance-dependence issues. For example, if I share my challenges with sobriety with a conservative, non-empathetic religious group (who may feel I have an addiction because of a moral failing), I feel no empathy and get no emotional relief. In fact, I would likely feel misunderstood, rejected, isolated and shamed. My stress level would increase, increasing my chance of relapse.

On the contrary, in AA meetings, I receive smiles, hugs and applause for achieving chronological milestones of sobriety. I am rewarded and "a part of." I feel good about myself, motivated to get more hugs and applause with the next chronological milestone. In an AA meeting, when I share my struggles with alcohol, I receive support; I perceive empathy. However, if I share my struggles with alcohol in a group of Overeaters Anonymous (OA) or even Narcotics Anonymous (NA), I perceive relatively less understanding and empathy than I would receive in a room of Alcoholics Anonymous (AA). Therefore, I find that OA and NA meetings are less effective in providing emotional healing and stress reduction than AA meetings for myself, a pure alcoholic. Similarly, an individual with a weight problem gets little benefit from sharing his or her distress with overeating in an AA meeting. This is why the written traditions of Twelve-Step groups emphasize a *"singleness of purpose."*

The empathy and confidentiality of a Twelve-Step group is reflected in the common-thread principle of all Twelve-Step groups: *anonymity.* With anonymity, there is protection from judgment from other people who may not be sympathetic or empathetic to the struggles of the substance-dependent. The Twelfth, and considered the most important, Tradition of all Twelve-Step groups reads: *"Anonymity is the spiritual foundation of all our traditions, ever reminding us to place principles before personalities"* (AA Twelve Steps and Twelve Traditions, p 184).

Anonymity and confidentiality ensures empathy. Positive, empathetic social interactions are associated with positive emotional states, which manifest themselves in a unified pattern of physiological and behavioral changes. Social interactions incorporate the exchange of emotional and physical energy. These interactions lead to physiological adaptations necessary for relaxation, digestion, anabolic metabolism, growth and healing. The corresponding mental states associated with positive social interactions include calmness and openness to social engagement.

To understand the biology of positive social interactions, it is useful to contrast such interactions with the more commonly studied defense reactions, such as the stress response associated with the "fight-or-flight" phenomenon, described by Cannon (1932). Although this subject was reviewed thoroughly in Chapter 5, a brief review is warranted. During the "fight-or-flight" response, the sympathetic (stimulatory) component of the autonomic nervous system is activated. There is an increase in cardiovascular activity, vascular dilation in the skeletal muscles, and an increase in respiratory rate. The hypothalamic-pituitary-adrenal axis is activated secreting corticotropin release factor (CRF) and cortisol. Cortisol, in synergy with catecholamines (adrenaline), results in increased glucose release from storage sites in the liver and muscles, increasing glucose metabolism. Concurrently, there is an inhibition of digestive and anabolic processes. At the same time, mental arousal and enhanced levels of aggression or fear (amygdala) may occur.

Although the animal (like man) in the "flight-or-flight" mode is agitated and "uncomfortable," these responses are evolutionarily adaptive: They force the animal to modify its environment to return to a more comfortable, homeostatic state. If your environment is causing you stress, you have either to "fight it" or "take flight." Unfortunately, as we discussed in Chapter 5, this stress state also catalyzes the use of mood-altering substances (a way of taking flight), which, under most circumstances, is maladaptive.

Through the positive emotions generated in association with positive social interactions, the antithesis of the stress response occurs. When one feels empathy, comfort, calm or "connectedness," there is a slight predominance of the parasympathetic (inhibitory) nervous system. The cardiovascular and respiratory systems are slowed. In an "energy-saving" mode, glucose is stored, rather than mobilized, and growth and healing can occur. The HPA axis is down regulated. Stress hormones, CRF, and cortisol are reduced and there is release of comfort hormones, such as oxytocin.

Several lines of evidence have pointed strongly to the central role of the small peptide, oxytocin, as a common regulatory element in feeling comfortable. Stimulated in the breast-feeding mother, it promotes maternal-infant bonding and provides a rewarding and relaxing response. Oxytocin has been called the "comfort" or the "tend-and-befriend" hormone. Oxytocin coordinates both the causes and effects of positive social interactions. During social interactions, oxytocin can be released by sensory stimuli perceived as positive, including touch, warmth, and odors. The consequences of positive social interactions, such as reduced sympathoadrenal activity and enhanced parasympathetic-vagal activity, are also partially mediated by oxytocin. *Because the release of oxytocin can become conditioned to emotional states and mental images, the actions of this peptide may provide an additional explanation for the long-term benefits of positive social experiences.*

It would be naive, however, to believe that a single hormone could be responsible for the antistress effects of positive social interactions and the mother-infant relationship. Other neurotransmitters (e.g., GABA, glutamate, serotonin, acetylcholine, nitric oxide, endorphin/opioid peptides, sex hormones, and endocannabinoids) may also play roles in social attachment physiology (Esch, 2002, Rodriguez, 1998). The following discussion serves to simplify our understanding of this emerging and relatively complex science.

What We Can Learn from Animal Populations

Edward O. Wilson is a Harvard biologist and Nobel Laureate for his work in animal sociobiology. When I sat in his lectures and in the latest edition of the summary of his life's work, *Sociobiology* (Wilson, 1975), he described the fundamentals of population density dynamics. Pertinent to our discussion is that mammals, when either isolated or in very densely populated environments are in a stressed condition, both individually and as a population. It is well-know that rats, when isolated, exhibit signs of stress: They lose weight, despite having adequate food, they become aggressive with their handlers and they have irregular sleep/wake schedules. Similarly, when rats are housed in densely populated cages with adequate food, they show signs of increased stress. they have high cortisol levels and suppressed immune function, lose weight, and do not reproduce despite ample mates (Veatch, 2008). Studies of deer populations have shown similar findings; however, they are even more elucidating.

Although, it is well-known that a high population density adversely affects deer weight gain and reproduction ability, it was generally thought to be due to food shortages. A study exploring the effects of high density on social stress in white–tailed deer was conducted in upper Michigan by researchers John J. Ozoga and Louis J. Verme (1985). These researchers generously fed an enclosed deer herd until it resembled a wild herd that exceeded the carrying capacity of the land. They provided unlimited feed and allowed it grow to ten times the acceptable carrying capacity (over 100 deer per square mile). Interestingly, the researchers found that as deer density increased the survival rate of fawns decreased. Keep in mind that access to high quality feed was unlimited. Ozoga states, "Density stress . . . independent of nutrition can alter a doe's rate of physical maturation and reproductive performance." There was a direct correlation between the fawning success of does and their social rank within the herd. Ozoga notes that, "neonatal mortality was due primarily to abandonment of fawns and imprinting failure as a result of territorial behavior at high densities." Ozoga concluded that the lack of fawn–rearing space for subordinate does resulted in higher fawn mortality. Given what we know from human and rodent data, I believe the fawn abandonment, lack of imprinting, and poor physical maturation, are due to poor fawn nurturing and, therefore, low oxytocin levels.

In the Michigan study, increasing deer density also affected antler development, a measure of sexual dimorphism (sexual differentiation). When the deer density was low, yearling bucks did not exhibit short spikes. However, at higher densities, 22 percent of the yearling bucks grew short spikes as their first set of antlers. Keep in mind that proper nutrition was available even as densities increased to ten times that which the natural habitat conditions could sustain. Ozoga and Verme concluded that, "socially stressed male fawns experienced a physiological setback and probable sex hormone imbalance that impaired antler development." While it is well documented that a lack of adequate nutrition will prevent a buck from reaching its full genetic potential, it is apparent that density-related social stress can produce similar effects. Biologists now believe that social stress may be affecting sexual dimorphism, antler growth and fawn recruitment in dense herds, and these effects are likely also due to low oxytocin levels.

It is easy to extrapolate these findings to observations made in human populations (Winsborough, 1965). We are well aware that prolonged social isolation, as well as prolonged exposure to high population density, induces stress (e.g., being stuck in a elevator or prison). What we learn from our animal studies is that the chronic hormonal changes under either of these circumstances can impair growth (anabolic processes), and neural development (Conrad, 2010).

The changes observed in deer populations are entirely socially and emotionally induced, due to the impairment of cooperative and empathetic affiliation and the promotion of aggressive, competitive interactions. These changes are likely specifically related to chronically elevated cortisol levels and suppressed oxytocin levels. Other neurotransmitters likely play important, but smaller roles. Most germane to our current topic, we know from animal and human studies, is that chronic stress or cortisone injections increases the risk for substance abuse (Apter, 2006, Chapter 5).

The Rewarding Nature of Positive Social Interaction

As addressed in previous chapters, the involvement of the mesocorticolimbic pathways in processing reward and addiction has been thoroughly studied in recent years. Evidence from animal studies or functional MR imaging studies in humans indicates that the reward circuit in the striatum and limbic system, mediated by dopamine, is involved in processing rewarding non-social stimuli, such as money, food, and psychostimulant drugs (Koob, 1997; Schultz, 1997; Knutson, 2001; Izuma, 2008).

It has been hypothesized that these same reward pathways have evolved to facilitate pro-social behaviors to facilitate reproduction and other evolutionarily adaptive social interactions (Kelley, 2002). Indeed, several empirical studies support this hypothesis and indicate that social r of various social stimuli that eward is processed in the same limbic reward circuits as non-social reward and drug addiction. Studies in rodents highlight the importance of striatal dopamine for highly socially motivated behavior such as maternal care, mating behavior and social attachment. For instance, the access to pups is more reinforcing than cocaine in female rats (Insel, 2003), and dopamine in the nucleus accumbens is involved in typical mating behavior and social interactions of monogamous prairie voles (Wang, 2004; Liu, 2010).

Data from functional MR imaging studies in humans exhibit striatal activations for a variety of rewarding social stimuli such as beautiful faces (Aharon, 2001), positive emotional expressions (Rademacher, 2010), one's own social reputation (Izuma, 2008) and maternal and romantic love (Bartels, 2000, 2004). A relatively recent study has shown activation of the nucleus accumbens, putamen, and thalamic nuclei during the anticipation of positive social feedback (Spreckelmeyer, 2009). Romantic love has been shown to activate the reward centers on function MRI exams (Saxe, 2008). However, this activation may not be as strong or enduring as that achievable by addictive drugs. *Because of their synthetic potency, drugs of abuse completely surpass normal physiology.*

Altogether, there is evidence from a variety of studies that the dopaminergic reward circuits form the primary neural system for processing rewards of various non-social stimuli that could motivate social behavior. A wealth of literature analyzing social behaviors indicate that processing of social stimuli is certainly more complicated than dopamine release in the striatum on its own. Other neurotransmitters, such as catecholamines, and neuropeptides, such as oxytocin and endorphins, and many others likely modulate activity in these neural circuits (Insel, 2003; Skuse, 2009). Pro-social behaviors are more than finding "reward," as in attaining "comfort" and reducing stress. As such, the social organism is complex.

At this point in the discussion, it is worthwhile to distinguish "reward" and "pleasure" from "comfort." The term "reward" can be ascribed to the limbic gratification one gets from food, sex, addictive drugs, money, or praise. Reward stimulates appetence, and appetence motivates behavior toward more reward. The limbic dopamine pathways of the brain offer the primary neural substrate of reward. "Pleasure," on the other hand, describes a "state or feeling of happiness or satisfaction resulting from an experience that one enjoys." Pleasure, therefore, has a more subjective connotation with cognitive, behavioral and motivational overtones. In neurobiology, pleasure refers to the cognitive satisfaction received from reward and motivation circuitries that are imbedded in the limbic system as well as in higher cortical centers. It is the "good feeling" that comes from behaviorally satisfying homeostatic needs such as hunger, sex, and overall bodily comfort. Reward and pleasure are modulated by dopamine.

"Comfort," however, is defined as "to soothe, console, or reassure." Comfort implies a reduction in stress, whereas reward and pleasure may co-exist with stress and frequently are not stress reducing. This is clearly the case in addiction, where reward and pleasure from mood-altering substances have little or no effect on stress and may actually promote it. In neurobiology, "comfort" is primarily modulated by the parasympathetic (inhibitory) division of the autonomic nervous system, endorphins and oxytocin. Oxytocin has been shown to reduce stress through reducing the reactivity of the HPA axis and promote maternal-infant and other types of social bonding.

The interaction of dopamine and oxytocin in social interactions has been studied in animal and human populations. Recent research has shown that simultaneous activation of dopaminergic reward and oxytocin pathways is critical to relationship formation (Skuse, 2008). Similarly, Depuea (2005) argued that oxytocin is implicated in both the motivation and the reward associated with social interactions beyond the mating arena. Their study showed that dopaminergic neurons running from the ventral tegmental area to the nucleus accumbens are responsible for the motivation to affiliate. They also showed that oxytocin and oxytocin receptors are found in these same areas and interact with the dopamine system. In addition, opioid peptides (e.g. morphine) have been shown to promote affiliative physiology, as are presumably the endorphins (Esch, 2004). Oxytocin can increase endorphin release by up to 300 percent (Csiffary, 1992).

Thus, although the following discussion will focus on the central role of oxytocin in stress reduction and social bonding, I caution the reader that other neurotransmitters are likely involved and the relationships between neural circuits are very complex, rife with biphasic responses, receptor competition and modification, inhibitory feedback loops, and the like. *In this context, I suspect there will be no "magic pill" or nasal mist that brings us the benefits of empathetic or affectionate relationships.*

Oxytocin, the "Comfort" Hormone

Oxytocin has been identified as the most common hormone implicated in the comfort, or "antistress," response. Recently, there has been a surge of interest in oxytocin which has spread swiftly from medical journals to the popular media. Its popularity owes much to the attractive terms used to describe its psychological effects, such as *love, trust,* and *bonding.* Although there is general agreement on oxytocin's prosocial effects, there are various suggestions about how these are mediated. Several lines of research in animals and humans support the facts that (1) oxytocin enhances attachment and trust and improves social memory and bonding, and (2) oxytocin reduces fear and stress.

Oxytocin is a peptide hormone composed of nine amino acids (Goodson, 2008; Lee, 2009). It is present in all mammalian species. Oxytocin has central and peripheral effects. Peripherally, oxytocin regulates uterine contractions during labor and milk ejection during lactation, and functions in sexual orgasm. It is synthesized in the magnocellular neurons of the paraventricular (PVN) and supraoptic (SON) nuclei of the hypothalamus, which project to the posterior pituitary where oxytocin is released into blood circulation. Centrally, oxytocin acts as a neuro-modulator. Released from all parts of the neuronal membrane, oxytocin diffuses widely, affecting many regions of the brain (Landgraf, 2004). Oxytocin receptors are found in many parts of the brain and spinal cord, including the amygdala, hypothalamus, septum, hippocampus, amygdala, striatum, hypothalamus, nucleus accumbens, and brainstem. Central oxytocin effects include maternal and sexual behavior, pair bonding, and social recognition (Donaldson, 2008).

Maternal Bonding and Antistress Effects of Oxytocin

Oxytocin was first identified in lactating females and is responsible for inducing uterine contractions in childbirth. Its role has been expanded to include promoting social attachment and stress reduction. The most enduring social bond is maternal-infant attachment. The tender intimacy and attachment of a mother for her infant, and vice versa, occupies a uniquely lauded position in human social behavior. Mother-infant attachment provides one of the most striking examples of social bonding and is worthy of review prior to discussing other forms of pro-social behaviors mediated by oxytocin.

Maternal breast-feeding and maternal-infant attachment represents examples of positive social interactions, which have been explored extensively in animals and humans. In order to facilitate the description of neuroendocrine mechanisms, this kind of interaction can be divided into different phases of activity. In the act of breast-feeding, a mother not only gives milk but also transmits warmth to her young by dilating the blood vessels in the skin overlying the mammary gland. Furthermore, the mother provides warmth, protection, and care. The mother also receives during breast-feeding. The suckling, touching, and warmth generated by the offspring activate maternal skin sensory nerve afferents, which results in milk ejection as well the other "giving" effects described above. Milk ejection is caused by smooth muscle (myoepithelial) contractions in the mammary gland and warmth is induced by vascular dilation in the breast—both effects mediated by oxytocin.

In addition to changes seen in lactation, oxytocin has been shown to produce acute as well as long-term relaxation or "antistress" behavioral effects in the mother (Uvna¨s-Moberg, 1996a, 1996b). Secondary to repeated exposure to the suckling stimulus, lactating rats demonstrate decreased sympathetic nervous tone, manifested as lowered blood pressure, when compared with non-lactating rats. They also have an enhanced vagal (parasympathetic) nerve tone, contributing to decreased heart rate and blood pressure. Increased vagal tone also leads to increased release of insulin and of other gastrointestinal hormones. Together, these results show a shift in autonomic nervous system tone from sympathetic (stimulatory or stressed) to parasympathetic (inhibitory or relaxed). Furthermore, lactating rats are less responsive to stressful external stimuli than are non-lactating animals (Uvna¨s-Moberg, 1996a, 1996b).

Similar antistress effects occur in breastfeeding women. Breast-feeding women demonstrate with each breastfeeding session a fall in blood pressure and cortisol levels, as well as a rise in plasma levels of gastrointestinal digestive hormones (Amico, 1994; Nissen, 1996; Uvna¨s-Moberg, 1996a).

There are a number of studies showing that the antistress effects seen with breast-feeding are mediated through oxytocin. Indeed, administration of oxytocin to both male and female rats exerts potent physiological antistress effects. After acute administration of oxytocin, a sedative effect is induced as exemplified in decreased locomotor activity (Uvna¨s-Moberg, 1994). After oxytocin administration, the withdrawal latency in response to heat and mechanical stress stimuli is prolonged (A°gren, 1995; Lundeberg, 1994), there is a release of gastrointestinal hormones including insulin (Bjorkstrand, 1996a, 1996b) and the temperature of the tail skin is lowered (A°gren, 1995). After oxytocin injection, cortisol levels and blood pressure decrease within a few hours (Uvna¨s-Moberg, 1997a, 1997b, 1998). If daily oxytocin injections are repeated over a five-day period, the antistress effects of oxytocin become even more pronounced. After chronic oxytocin exposure, blood pressure is decreased by 10–20 mm-Hg (Petersson, 1996a) the withdrawal latency to heat (painful) stimuli is prolonged (Petersson, 1996b), cortisol levels are decreased and insulin and cholecystokinin levels are increased. In these animal experiments, the researchers noted that the effects last from one to several weeks after the last injection (Uvna¨s-Moberg 1997a, 1997b, 1998).

In humans, several studies have looked at the personality profiles of breast-feeding women. Breast-feeding women become more social, calm, and more tolerant to monotony. Oxytocin levels are positively correlated with scores obtained on personality tests reflecting social competency and calmness; this finding supports the hypothesis that oxytocin may play a role in these psychological adaptations (Nissen, 1998; Uvna¨s-Moberg, 1990).

In breast-feeding women, the analysis of correlations between oxytocin levels and personality traits, as determined by personality inventories, indicated that increased levels of social interaction, and decreased levels of anxiety correlated with different phases of oxytocin release. For example, the number of oxytocin pulses occurring in response to breastfeeding correlated with openness to social interactions, while basal oxytocin levels correlated with calmness. The number of oxytocin pulses and the openness to social interactions also correlated with the amount of milk given by the mother. Thus, a pulsatile oxytocin release pattern was associated with both psychological and physical components of the oxytocin-induced pro-social behaviors. The researchers concluded that the increased levels of calm are reflective of the "antistress" effects of oxytocin (Nissen, 1996, 1998).

As described in Chapter 5, the noradrenergic (stimulatory) system emanating from the locus ceruleus (LC) nucleus in the brainstem plays an important role in arousal and vigilance associated with stress. Stimulation of the noradrenergic system has been further associated with the suppression of emotionality, social competence, and pro-social behaviors (Henry, 1993a). These activating effects of noradrenaline are mediated by stimulation of a variety of receptors belonging to subclasses of adrenergic receptors (Nicholas, 1996). Oxytocin has been shown to moderate the activity of one of these adrenergic receptors to reduce blood pressure. Recently, oxytocin also has been shown to enhance the ability of clonidine, an adrenergic agonist, to inhibit firing of noradrenergic LC neurons (Uvna, 1998). Because the personality profile of breastfeeding women is characterized by increased social competence and calmness, this profile may be regarded as an antithesis to the behavioral pattern of the fight-or-flight response. Because the fight-or-flight response reflects a strong LC activation (Henry, 1993b), researchers have speculated that the psychological as well as physiological antistress effects of oxytocin may be related to modulating adrenergic receptor activity in the central nervous system.

In addition to its lactating and antistress physiological effects, oxytocin has been shown to promote bonding between ewe and lamb (Kendrick, 1987). Rodent studies have explored the possibility that pair bonding might similarly be associated with oxytocin release, an expectation arising from the proposal that adult attachment may have arisen from the more primitive mechanism of mother-infant bonding (Witt, 1992; Neuman, 2003). Two closely related species provided a convenient natural experiment (Insel, 1992). The prairie vole shows a strong partner preference and biparental care in contrast to the promiscuous montane vole. In the female prairie vole, oxytocin administration facilitates partner preference, whereas oxytocin antagonists block it, without interfering with mating. In the prairie vole, oxytocin receptors are found in the nucleus accumbens and perilimbic cortex, areas rich in dopamine receptors, as in humans. In these animals, administration of oxytocin induces central dopamine release and vice versa, and their synergistic action appears to be critical for partner preference (Edwards, 2006; Liu, 2003; Young, 2004). In the promiscuous montane vole, the oxytocin and dopamine systems are uncoupled, unlike humans.

In humans, evidence for maternal-fetal bonding associated with oxytocin has come from studies that assayed plasma oxytocin levels during the first and third trimester of pregnancy and the first post partum month. In one study, a pattern of increasing oxytocin during pregnancy was associated with higher maternal-fetal bonding (Levine, 2007). In another study, oxytocin levels in early pregnancy and postpartum were significantly correlated with maternal bonding measures, including attachment related thoughts, gaze at the infant, affectionate touch, and frequent infant checking (Feldman, 2007). The study by Dr. Feldman measured plasma levels of oxytocin in sixty-two pregnant women at three points: during the first trimester, the third trimester and the first month postpartum. The research team found that women with higher levels of oxytocin in the first trimester bonded better with their babies. It also found that those with higher oxytocin levels throughout the entire pregnancy and in the first month postpartum reported more behaviors that supported the formation of an exclusive relationship with their babies, such as singing special songs or bathing and feeding their infants in specific ways.

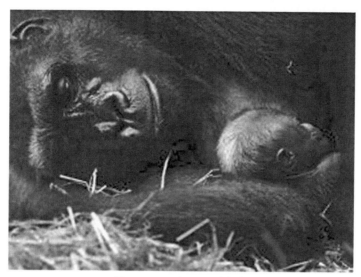

Happy mother and baby

The Antistress Effects of Oxytocin in Non-Mother-Infant Relations

The antistress effects of oxytocin are uniformly recognized in human and animal research. Animal studies have shown that administering oxytocin reduces amygdala activation, increases parasympathetic functioning, inhibits corticotropin-releasing factor neurons, decreases corticosteroid release, and results in lower levels of fearful behavior (Engelmann, 2004; Neumann, 2007; Viviani, 2008). Oxytocin activates neurons in the lateral and capsular portion of the central amygdala, which inhibit, via GABA projections, the fear-inducing effects of vasopressin in the medial central amygdala (Huber, 2005).

Functional MRI studies of humans during oxytocin administration have produced interesting and positive findings. In response to fear-provoking visual stimuli, oxytocin reduced amygdala activation and the connectivity between the amygdala and the upper brainstem in the region of the locus ceruleus, the region implicated in autonomic nervous system reactions to threat (Kirsch, 2005). Petrovic (2008) fear-conditioned his humans to a set of faces using electric shock while being shown certain faces. After oxytocin treatment, the fear-conditioned group showed reduced activity in the amygdala and anterior medial temporal cortex (the area around the amygdala) and in the anterior cingulate cortex (perilimbic cortex, attention). When fear-conditioned faces displayed direct gaze (taken to be the most threatening), activity in the amygdala was significantly higher than in the placebo group and attenuated with oxytocin. The oxytocin group also showed a significant attenuation in their affective (subjective emotional) ratings of the fear-conditioned faces. Another study (Domes, 2007) found that oxytocin eliminated the heightened amygdala activation seen in the placebo group to emotional versus neutral faces. Interestingly, this effect was seen for happy as well as sad and fearful faces, suggesting that oxytocin effects may not be specific to fear reduction, but rather to generalized heightened affective stimuli.

Other studies have administered oxytocin prior to stress manipulation to examine possible antistress effects. In a study by Dr. Ditzen, from the University of Zurich, romantic-couple subjects were asked to discuss an area of conflict in their relationship (designed to induce stress). Post-discussion cortisol levels were significantly lower in those couples who had previously received oxytocin (Ditzen, 2009). The separate and joint effects of oxytocin and social support on stress reactivity were examined by Heinrichs (2003). The experimental design compared four groups resulting from pharmacological condition (oxytocin or placebo administration) and presence or absence of social support (participants brought a friend who accompanied them during the ten-minute preparation period prior to a public speech). *Social support was more effective than oxytocin in attenuating cortisol response, but the lowest cortisol reactivity was seen in those participants receiving both social support and oxytocin.* A comparison of pre- and post-stress anxiety levels showed that oxytocin significantly reduced self-reported anxiety.

The Prosocial Effects of Oxytocin in Non-Mother-Infant Relations

Oxytocin is known to stimulate sexual behavior in rats and has been shown to be released in response to sexual interactions in both rats and humans (Carter, 1998) It is possible, therefore, that oxytocin is involved in some of the physiological and behavioral adaptations that occur during sexual behavior (Carter, 1992). Other researchers have identified roles for oxytocin and dopamine in interpersonal attraction, considering the simultaneous activation of dopaminergic reward and oxytocin pathways to be critical to relationship formation (Skuse, 2008). Beyond the mating arena, Depue (2005) argues that oxytocin is implicated in both the motivation and the reward associated with social interactions.

Animal studies suggest that it may be implicated in general sociability. Bonnet monkeys, a naturally affiliative species, show higher oxytocin levels in cerebrospinal fluid than the less sociable pigtail macaque (Rosenblum, 2002). In rats, gerbils, and squirrel monkeys, intracranial or subcutaneous injection of oxytocin increases social contact time (Razzoli, 2003). Within species, individual differences in affiliation may reflect early nurturing experiences and their effects on the oxytocin system (Cushing, 2005). Rhesus monkeys deprived of maternal care display antisocial behavior, including avoidance of physical contact and gaze, stereotypical and self-directed behaviors, and attachment to inanimate objects. These monkeys also have decreased cerebrospinal oxytocin measured between eighteen and thirty-six months. Levels of cerebrospinal oxytocin (but not plasma oxytocin) are positively correlated with affiliative behavior (Winslow, 2005).

A number of researchers have proposed that the prosocial effect of oxytocin is derived from its antistress properties. Oxytocin, by reducing interpersonal fear or anxiety, allows for the formation of positive bonds. Administration of oxytocin increases ratings of trustworthiness and attractiveness of unfamiliar faces in both men and women (Theodoridou, 2009). Tops (2007) found a positive correlation between oxytocin and attachment as measured by the tendency to express and share emotions and feelings with others. Grewen (2005) found that individuals who reported a more supportive relationship with their partner had higher oxytocin levels throughout a series of three blood draws taken before, during, and after warm partner contact. Taylor (2006) proposed that elevated oxytocin levels act as a marker for gaps in relationships (perhaps due to the stress of loneliness) and trigger a search for affiliative contact.

Somatosensory Stimulation and Oxytocin: The Massage Factor

It is known that breastfeeding or suckling releases maternal oxytocin levels through somatosensory (skin) stimulation. However, oxytocin may also be released by non-noxious activation of somatosensory neurons in general, in males as well as females. In rats, studies have shown that several types of non-noxious stimuli—such as touch, warm temperature, vibration, and electro-acupuncture— increase oxytocin levels in plasma and particularly in cerebrospinal fluid (Stock and Uvna¨s-Moberg, 1988; Uvna¨s-Moberg, 1993). In conscious rats, massage-like stroking of the abdomen is also followed by increased oxytocin levels (A°gren, 1995). Therefore, oxytocin also is likely to be released in response to activation of somatosensory afferents caused by social contact and grooming. Non-noxious stimulation—such as that induced experimentally by low-intensity electrical stimulation, brushing of the leg in anesthetized rats, or stroking the abdomen—lowers blood pressure, decreases electrical activity in the sympathoadrenal nerve, and lowers levels of plasma catecholamines and cortisol.

Physical therapies, including massage, have been shown to reduce anxiety and lower cortisol levels in humans (Field, 1992; Gonzalez, 1994). Massage also releases oxytocin in both humans (Rapaport, 2010) and animals (A°gren, 1995). In addition, comparable somatosensory stimulation increases activity in the vagal nerve, as reflected, for example, by the release of gastrointestinal hormones (Araki, 1984; Kurosawa, 1982, 1985; Uvna¨s-Moberg, 1986, 1992). In humans, massage elevates oxytocin (Zach, 200x) lowers blood pressure (Kurosawa et al., 1995) and stimulates a release of vagally-regulated gastrointestinal hormones (Uvna¨s-Moberg et al., 1992), indicating a shift from sympathetic to parasympathetic autonomic dominance. In addition, rats that have received massage show withdrawal latency to heat, mechanical stimuli is prolonged, and tail-skin temperature is reduced (A°gren, 1995). Furthermore, after massage, animals (and humans) appear mildly sedated as reflected by reduced locomotor behavior (Uvna¨s-Moberg, 1996a, 1996b).

The Physiology of Trust and Empathy

In humans, the experience of being trusted and reciprocating trust is associated with raised oxytocin levels. Zak, Kurzban, and Matzner (2005) used a simple Trust Game in which an investor awarded a sum of money (between one and ten dollars) to a trustee that was tripled in value by the experimenter. In a control condition, the amount awarded to the trustee was decided by a random computer draw. In the subsequent experimental condition, plasma oxytocin levels in the trustee were significantly higher. The authors suggested that the trustees' oxytocin levels were responsive to the intention of trust rather than to the receipt of money per se. The amount returned to the investor (a measure of trustworthiness) was significantly correlated with subsequent oxytocin levels for experimental, but not control participants. It is noteworthy that, given that oxytocin appears to be secreted in times of trust, as well as its antistress and anabolic effects, oxytocin has been implicated in the "placebo effect."

In a similar trust game (Kosfeld, 2005), the researchers concluded that the higher level of trust after oxytocin administration was caused by a decrease in betrayal aversion and social avoidance. Interacting with a stranger, whose reputation and past behavior are unknown to us, is normally associated with a degree of apprehension. This research group found that this apprehension is decreased by oxytocin, thereby permitting trust. Another study (Baumgartner and Heinrichs, 2008) examined the impact of a breach of trust on trusting behavior by the investor. After being informed that the trustee had repaid them on only 50 percent of occasions, the placebo group showed a decrease in trusting behavior (reduced money transfer) accompanied by increased activation in the amygdala and brainstem, changes not seen in the oxytocin group. These results support the hypothesis that oxytocin reduces fear and conserves trust even in situations of betrayal.

Combining the research approaches of previous studies of somatosensory stimulation and trust, Morhenn (2008) examined their joint effects on changes in plasma oxytocin while performing a trust game. Participants received a fifteen-minute massage or rested before playing the Trust Game (a third group received the massage only). Blood draws for oxytocin assays took place on arrival and at the end of the experiment. For the investors, there was no association between the sum of money they transferred ("trust") and change in oxytocin levels either with or without prior massage. But for those trustees who had received the massage, there was a significant positive association between the sum received (reflective of "trustworthiness") and an increase in their oxytocin level. The amount returned by the trustee to the investor was also correlated with oxytocin change both with and without massage. Because massage alone did not alter oxytocin levels, the authors suggest that it is touch associated with being trusted that induces oxytocin elevation.

Eye gaze toward different facial features in photographs was used as an assay of social interest by Guastella (2008). Compared with placebo, oxytocin increased the duration and frequency of men's gaze toward the eyes. The eyes can convey information about a target's emotional state, and this has formed the basis for a measure of empathy called the Reading the Mind in the Eyes test (Baron-Cohe, 2001). Oxytocin increased the correct identification of emotions with the effect being more marked on the most difficult items (Domes, 2007).

In an experimental paradigm designed to study "empathy," Zak (2007) compared the effect of oxytocin on two economic games. In the Ultimatum Game, one player is assigned a sum of money to be split with another participant. If the offer is accepted, the money is paid to both participants, as agreed, but if the offer is rejected, both parties receive nothing. This game is taken as a measure of perspective taking (because the donor must consider what offer the other party is likely to accept). In the Dictator Game, one player decides how much of the assigned sum to award to the second party, which the second party has no option but to accept. The authors reported that oxytocin administration significantly increased the money awarded in the Ultimatum Game but not in the Dictator Game, suggesting that the effect of oxytocin is on empathy-mediated generosity rather than generous behavior per se. This conclusion is consistent with on performed by Kosfeld (2005), in which, following oxytocin or placebo administration, participants played the Trust Game described earlier. Oxytocin increased the value of money transferred by the investor, supporting its role in enhancing trusting behavior, although it did not affect subjective ratings of interpersonal trust. The study further showed that oxytocin had no effect on the back transfer of money by the trustee, suggesting that oxytocin does not have a generalized effect on reciprocity or generosity in the absence of a requirement to empathize with another's perspective.

One can conclude from these studies that oxytocin facilitates empathy, and the effect of oxytocin on prosocial behavior is most evident when an individual must take into account another's perspective. Romantic relationships, associated with oxytocin release, involve continual monitoring of another's perspective (Fisher, 2006; Zeki, 2007), and human mothering involves maternal empathetic connection with the infant (Meins, 2001). By lowering perceived threat and increasing trust, oxytocin appears to facilitate empathetic identification.

Stress Promotes Social Interaction and Bonding: Seeking Comfort

Indeed, it is easy to suggest from the literature that the effect of oxytocin is not to promote trust, but rather reduce fear. *The most consistent and pervasive empirical finding in the literature on oxytocin is that it depresses amygdala activity and HPA stress responses and that this reduction is linked to stronger social approach behavior.* Evidence for attachment formation comes from behavioral changes associated with mammalian birth, lactation, and sexual interactions (Carter, 1998). Mammalian birth is clearly a stressful experience. In the mother, physiological events preceding and accompanying parturition involve exceptionally high levels of adrenal activity and the release of various peptides, including endogenous opioid peptides, oxytocin, and vasopressin (Keverne, 1992). As mentioned before, stressful experiences or challenges may encourage increased social behaviors and attachment (Carter, 1998).

Hence, comparatively high levels of HPA axis activity or other indicators of stressor-sympathetic arousal, and a subsequent release of oxytocin, have been measured under conditions that commonly precede or are associated with the formation of social bonds. These bonds may buffer against stress, facilitating social support, security, and closeness, since the presence of a partner may provide a social form of stress relief (Esch, 2003). *Taken together, positive social behaviors, including social bonds, reduce HPA axis activity and stress.* The central action of oxytocin, therefore, has been implicated in both social bonding and the central dampening/control of the HPA axis (Carter, 1998). Threatening or challenging situations encourage the return to a secure base or otherwise strengthen social bonds (Parnskepp, 1997). Oxytocin, however, is capable of inducing positive social behaviors, and both oxytocin and social interactions decrease activity in the HPA axis (i.e., stress) (DeVries, 1997; Esch, 2002a; 2002b; 2002c). Social interactions and attachments then activate endocrine or auto regulatory signaling systems that are able to further reduce stress (i.e., HPA hyper-reactivity), yet modulate emotions and the related autonomic nervous system's involvement, thereby, perhaps, accounting for health benefits that are attributed to social bonding (Heinrichs, 2003; Morhenn, 2008; Zak, 2005).

On a continuum of interpersonal perception, trust and fear reside at opposite extremes. Trust indicates a belief in the reliability and goodwill of another person and can range from provisional favorability to complete confidence. Fear signals threat, hostility, and possible attack and can range from mild apprehension to outright panic. These are not merely semantic distinctions. The behavioral manifestation of oxytocin's antistress action may depend on where an individual is located on this interpersonal continuum between trust and fear. It may downgrade terror to fear or shift mild apprehension to unconditional trust.

Studies that have manipulated central oxytocin in the context of economic games have shown that oxytocin increases trust, empathy, and generosity toward strangers. After acts of trust are betrayed by a stranger, oxytocin prevents the normal decline in trusting behavior (Baumgartner, 2008). This suggests that oxytocin increase the positivity of interactions in general, and its effect does not depend on a prior relationship between the parties (Theodoridou, 2009). I suggest that this positivity results from a decrease in the wariness with which we typically approach strangers.

More Meetings = More Empathetic Social Support = Less Stress

Oxytocin has emerged as a core component of the mechanisms mediating the health benefits and antistress effects of positive social interactions. Positive social behaviors and social bonding are characterized by repeated physical and emotional stimuli. As described above, each of these stimuli can reduce sympathoadrenal activity and increase parasympathetic-vagal activity and are capable of releasing oxytocin.

Both oxytocin and positive experiences can increase anabolic metabolism and, in some circumstances, growth and behavioral calmness. It is important to note that the antistress effects of oxytocin become more pronounced after repeated exposures. Social bonds also lead to repeated exposures to social stimuli and to the repeated release of oxytocin. Thus, individuals living within a social bond or supportive social group would be likely to be exposed to repetitive oxytocin release. Socially released oxytocin would induce a physiological state characterized by decreased sympathoadrenal and enhanced parasympathetic-vagal activity. Based on our understanding of oxytocin, this state would be characterized by calmness and reduced psychological reactivity to stressful or painful experiences.

In humans, social support and positive experiences have well-documented health benefits (Ryff, 1998; Shumaker, 1994). A good marriage and access to a supportive social network reduced the risk of several diseases, especially those associated with cardiovascular function and blood pressure. The finding that chronic oxytocin elevation is capable of producing long-term reductions in blood pressure and heart rate (Petersson, 1996a), provides one mechanism through which social support could directly benefit health (Uvna¨s-Moberg, 1997a, 1997b, 1998).

In my journey of recovery, I have found another family: the fellowship of Alcoholics Anonymous. I have an established home group of about one-hundred members, which is part of the broader fellowship of one million in the United States and over two million worldwide. I can travel anywhere in the world and socialize with individuals empathetic to my condition. In my home group, we all know each other by name, exchange numbers and Facebook addresses, and have a Yahoo group and a softball team. They are the most genuine people I know. We meet every day at 6:30 am to share our "experience, strength, and hope." An hour later, we adjourn, and I am off to work, into the world reeling with *stress*. I am ready now, with the fellowship behind me. No worries: My cell phone has a dozen phone numbers of recovering alcoholics at my fingertips.

Role of the Therapy Dog

There was a recent article in the Wall Street Journal written by Melinda Beck about a small but growing number of mental health professionals bringing their dogs to work in their private practices, where they help calm patients down, cheer them up and offer a happy distraction with a wagging tail. It is commonplace for a therapy dog to visit hospitals or nursing homes. The Betty Ford Center has a therapy dog named—well, of course, that's anonymous. Beck reports that these mental health professionals use these "canine therapy-assistants" who often work full days and get to know the patients just as well as the doctors.

In her article, Beck refers to patients who sometimes speak to the therapy dog, rather than to the psychotherapist, and patients can hug the dog, but not the therapist. She refers to accounts of patients in therapy and how the dogs provide comfort. In her article, Beck quotes Rebecca Johnson, who teaches a popular course in animal-human interaction at the University of Missouri, as saying: "It's chemical, not magical." Beck refers to research that I have not reviewed, which shows that a few minutes of stroking a pet dog decreases cortisol, the stress hormone, in both the human and the dog. It also increases prolactin and oxytocin, hormones that govern nurturing and security, as well as serotonin and norepinephrine, neurotransmitters that boost mood.

Beck quoted a marriage and family therapist in Los Alamitos, California, who practices with her eleven-year-old King Charles Spaniel, Duke, who she calls "a seeing heart dog," because Duke lies on the floor next to patients with anxiety disorders, and sits on the couch close to those who are depressed. It was reported that, on one occasion, Duke jumped up and sat next to a patient she had not realized was depressed before the patient opened his mouth. When the patient began to share, a swell of depression emanated.

Comfort Music

It is well known that pleasurable music can have calming effects on the listener. There have been a number of recent functional MRI studies showing that pleasurable music stimulates deep limbic structures, with a left-sided predominance (Altenmuller, 2001, 2002; Salamon, 2003). This is in contrast to the more negative perceptions following activations in right hemispheric structures in the amygdala, related to anxiety or fear. These findings are similar to those found with meditation, which also has been shown to increase left-sided anterior activation of the brain, as measurable by various EEG techniques (Esch, 2004). Davidson (2000, 2003) suggested that this particular brain activity pattern is associated with faster recovery and more adaptive responding to negative and/or stressful events (i.e., higher flexibility, stress reduction) (Davidson, 2000, 2003; Esch, 2003, 2004).

A study by Dr. Nilsson of the Department of Cardiothoracic Surgery and Centre for Health Care Sciences, Orebro University, Sweden, studied the effects of bed-rest combined with relaxing music for patients who have undergone heart surgery on postoperative day one (Nilsson, 2009). In the music group, levels of oxytocin increased significantly in contrast to the control group for which the trend over time was negative (i.e., decreasing values). Subjective relaxation levels increased significantly more, and there were significantly higher levels of arterial oxygen, implying improved respiration and cardiovascular tone, in the music group compared with the control group. The authors concluded that listening to music during bed rest after open-heart surgery has some effects on the relaxation system as regards s-oxytocin and subjective relaxations levels. This effect seems to have a causal relation from the psychological (music makes patients relaxed) to the physical (oxytocin release).

Altruism and Recovery

One of the foundations of Twelve Step recovery is the Twelfth Step itself which calls for the newly recovered alcoholic to get into service and to share his experience with others who are still suffering. In the rooms of AA, and all Twelve Step groups, there is a cry to the newcomer. The fellowship seeks out those who need help. *"Working with others"* has been the bedrock of Alcoholics Anonymous for decades, and many have benefited from its service. *"Unity, Service, and Recovery"* are written on the three sides of the AA triangle and are inscribed on all AA coins. *Altruism is fundamental to recovery and is socially and evolutionarily adaptive.*

In most cases, altruism stems from empathy, but that is not always the case. Not all altruistic behavior requires empathy. When animals alert others to an outside threat, work together for immediate reward, or vocally attract others to discovered food, biologists may speak of altruism or cooperation, but this behavior is unlikely to be motivated by empathy with the beneficiary. A flock of birds taking off all at once because one among them is startled shows a reflex-like, highly adaptive spreading of fear that may not involve any understanding of what triggered the initial reaction. Similarly, when a room full of human newborns bursts out crying because one among them started to cry, there is an automatic spreading of distress (Hoffman 1975). At the core of these processes is adoption of another's emotional state (i.e., emotional contagion) (Hatfield, 1993).

Emotional contagion, which may be otherwise termed self-centered vicarious arousal or distress, represents the oldest kind of empathy. Another good example is the intensified pain response of mice seeing other mice in pain (Langford, 2006). Emotional contagion may lead individuals frightened by the alarm of others to hide or flee, a mother distressed by her offspring's distress to reassure both herself and her offspring by warming or nursing them, or inhibit an individual from inflicting pain upon another because of the vicarious negative arousal induced by the other's distress calls. Thus, simple empathetic reactions may benefit both the actor and individuals close to them. Emotional contagion on a less dramatic level is the basis of cooperative behavior. Imagine a group of animals in which every member was to eat, sleep, forage, or play independently. This would be impossible for nomadic animals, such as primates and humans. Being empathetic and coordinated is often a matter of life or death; it is adaptive (Bonsai and Garber 2000).

Directed altruism requires the addition of other-orientation to emotional activation. In nonhuman primates, the most common empathy-based concern for others is defense against aggression. Exceptional urgency and extreme motivation are required because their action needs to be swift, and actors may face bodily danger when assisting others against an attacker. For example, when a female reacts to the screams of her closest associate by defending her against a dominant male, she takes enormous risk on behalf of the other.

In 1990, Jane Goodall wrote: *"In some zoos, chimpanzees are kept on man-made islands, surrounded by water-filled moats . . . Chimpanzees cannot swim and, unless they are rescued, will drown if they fall into deep water. Despite this, individuals have sometimes made heroic efforts to save companions from drowning—and were sometimes successful. One adult male lost his life as he tried to rescue a small infant whose incompetent mother had allowed it to fall into the water."* (Goodall, 1990, p. 213)

Admittedly, chimpanzees may deliberately engage in grooming as a way of gaining future return favors (Koyama, 2006), but grooming is a low-cost service. I do not see the chimp performing an economic risk/ benefit analysis of the situation of his compatriot floundering in the water. The chimp that quickly jumps in the water to save another must have an overwhelming immediate motivation, which is likely "emotional" or reward center-driven. The altruistic behavior was evolutionarily adaptive. Indeed, there is a wealth of systematic data on primate altruism, such as support in aggressive contexts (Harcourt and Deal, 1992), cooperation (Appealer and van Schawk, 2006), and food-sharing (Feistier & McGraw, 1989). Although some have argued that food-sharing may not be truly altruistic because it is subject to social pressure (Glibly, 2006), the problem with this view is that top-ranking individuals (who have no trouble resisting pressure) are among the most generous (Deal 1989), and sharing occurs even when individuals are separated by bars—hence insulated from pressure (de Waal 1997c, Nissan and Crawford 1932). *The actions, calls and begging of the hungry or injured induce empathy in the giver, who then returns altruistic behaviors.* Animals "know" that altruism is evolutionarily adaptive for the population.

Altruistic behavior has been described for cetaceans since the ancient Greeks. Dolphins are said to save companions by biting through harpoon lines or by hauling them out of nets in which they were entangled. Dolphins also support sick companions near the surface to keep them from drowning, and stay close females in labor. Whales tend to interpose themselves between a hunter's boat and injured conspecifics, or capsize the boat (Caldwell, 1966; Connor and Norris1982). Elephants are known to reassure distressed companions (Payne, 1998; Poole, 1996) and to support or lift up others too weak to stand (Hamilton-Douglas, 2006, Jobber 1991). For great apes, there exist literally hundreds of qualitative accounts of altruistic behaviors.

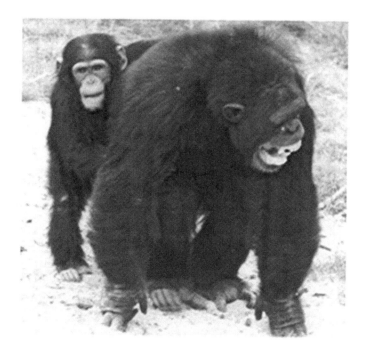

Consolation is common in humans and apes. Here a juvenile chimpanzee puts an arm around a screaming adult male, who has just been defeated in a fight. (from De Waal, 2008, with permission)

Animals are very empathetic, as it is in their own best interest to know the feelings of those around them; it is adaptive. They employ all their senses to perceive the intentions and feelings of others, as do humans. They employ sight to learn from subtle facial and body expressions, ears to learn from subtle vocalizations, and smell to detect whatever pheromone we do not know about or cannot measure. *Millions of years of evolution have shaped the lives of animals to survive, so if we learn from them, maybe we can, too.*

Proof of the "Joy of Giving"

Many ask the question: why are humans altruistic? An easy answer is that when we help someone in need, we expect him to return the favor. But some kinds of altruism cannot be explained by the weight of their reciprocity. For example, tax incentives aside, donating money to a charitable cause is unlikely to bring the donor any foreseeable return, except perhaps the *"joy of giving."*

Jorge Moll and Jordan Grafman, neuroscientists at the National Institutes of Health and LABS-D'Or Hospital Network provided the first evidence for the neural bases of "the joy of giving" in normal healthy human volunteers, using functional MR imaging. In their research, published in the Proceedings of the National Academy of Sciences (USA) in October 2006, they showed that both pure monetary rewards and charitable donations activated the mesolimbic reward pathway, a primitive part of the brain that usually lights up in response to food and sex (Moll, 2006).

Dr. Moll's study involved about twenty people, each of whom had the potential to walk away with a pot of $128. They also were given a separate pool of funds, which they could choose to distribute to a variety of charities linked to controversial issues, such as abortion and the death penalty. A computer presented each charity to the subjects in series and gave them the option to donate, to oppose donation, or to receive a payoff, adding money to the pot. Sometimes, the decision to donate or oppose was costly, calling for subjects to take money out of the pot.

It turned out that a similar pattern of brain activity was seen when subjects chose to either donate or take a payoff. Both types of decisions were associated with heightened activity in parts of the midbrain, a region deep in the brain that is known to be involved in primal desires (such as food and sex) and the satisfaction of them. *This result provides the first evidence that the "joy of giving" has an anatomical basis in the brain—surprisingly, one that is shared with selfish rewards, such as food, sex, and mood-altering substances.*

When volunteers generously placed the interests of others before their own by making charitable donations, another brain circuit was selectively activated: the subgenual cortex and septal regions of the extended reward center. These structures are intimately related to social attachment and bonding in other species. *Altruism, the experiment suggested, was not a superior moral faculty that suppresses basic selfish urges but rather was basic to the brain, hard-wired and pleasurable.*

Meanwhile, a study performed by Drs. Tankersley and Huettel, neuroscientists at Duke University Medical Center in Durham, North Carolina, connects altruism to the posterior superior temporal cortex (pSTC), an area in the upper rear of the brain that is known to enable us to perceive goal-directed actions by someone or something else. Among subjects who scored high on the altruism scale, the pSTC became more active during "watching" sessions and less active during "playing" sessions. Moreover, this link between pSTC activation and watching was strongest when the charity, not the subject, was designated to receive the game's winnings. Among low-altruism subjects, pSTC activation was not significantly altered by the conditions of the game—that is, whether the subject played or watched, and who received the winnings.

The authors suggest that the results show that altruism depends on, and may have evolved from, the brain's ability to perform the relatively low-level perceptual task of attributing actions to others. The authors further state that the findings are consistent with a theory that some aspects of altruism arose out of a system for perceiving the intentions and goals of others. Although his study and Dr. Moll's study link altruism to different brain regions, Dr. Huettel sees the results as complementary rather than contradictory. "There are certain to be multiple mechanisms that contribute to altruism, both in individuals and over evolutionary time," he said. From my own experience, as an altruistic individual and neuroradiologist, I agree that these studies are both accurate and complementary, and they prove to us as complex Homo sapiens what is instinctual and natural to our animal relatives.

What Do Apes Have to Do with Recovery?

Throughout this book, I have used several animal examples, particularly primates, to illustrate various points. We humans are too complicated to "get it" sometimes. This is certainly a failing of my own. I have never met an ape who read Aristotle or Plato, or had to think about the tax advantages of caring for his young. *We humans often lose sight of what is natural, beautiful, and right.* We can learn much from our animal friends.

We humans spend an inordinate amount of time either working too hard and thinking too little or working too little and thinking too hard.

I am guilty of both. We spend many turns of the clock and calendar contemplating, philosophizing, pontificating, and 'religionizing' about 'what is right and wrong.' We discuss morals and ethics ad nauseam. There are exhaustive ethics curricula at most universities. (This is not to suggest our study of morals and ethics is time wasted.)

We do have to recognize, however, that species lower on the phylogenetic tree, with a neocortex less than half the volume of ours, "do the right thing" because it is natural and rewarding at the most rudimentary level, their limbic brains. They have exactly the same limbic systems as we do, just a little smaller. The only difference between them and us is the size of our neocortex. The voluminous human neocortex is as much a curse, as it is a blessing. Are we truly "wise men" as our species name, Homo sapiens, suggests? If apes can 'do the right thing' and act 'selflessly' because it is in their biological nature, I cannot bear to hear my own excuse when I fail to do the same.

Some of us are consumed by self-centered and self-serving pursuits that make us lose sight of 'doing the right thing.' Serving an addictive habit is the prime example of selfishness and self-centeredness, as the authors of the *Big Book* remark numerous times. I see selfishness as the root cause of many evils, if not all. (Again, I am guilty.)

I sometimes ask myself the question: *Do apes know God?* The biologist in me says likely not. However, the faithful in me says that the apes and other social mammals 'do the right thing' because they are designed by a singular benevolent creator whose selflessness is apparent in numerous religious teachings. I do not really know. I can only observe behaviors and infer their motives. Most importantly, *I can truly only monitor my own behavior and make sure it is on the motivational plane of spiritual principles promoting selflessness and regard for others.* This is good for the planet. This is good for my recovery from addiction. The authors of the *Big Book* say so. The *"God of my understanding"* tells me so in numerous examples of His creation.

> *Why else are we here, if not to help one another.*
> ~Paul MacLean

Summary

Addiction is due to a dysfunctional, substance-dependent reward system, and is characterized by a stress state and cognitive impairment. Once an addict takes a drink or drug, the brain's limbic reward centers are activated strongly while, concurrently, the stress-response is activated and decision-making centers in the frontal lobe shut down. The body is reacting to a foreign substance that disrupts the nervous system. There is elevation of the stress hormone, cortisol, and a generalized increase in the activity of the excitatory nervous system, particularly in withdrawal states and in reaction to life stress. There is associated cognitive decline characterized by poor decision-making and judgement.

By comparing illustrations of the results of brain imaging studies, we see that areas activated by emotions (p. 84) are nearly identical to those activated by cravings (p. 115), <u>deactivated</u> in withdrawal and chronic use (p. 120), and responsible for cognitive impairment (p. 163).

Our emotional cognitive controls and maturity are arrested as natural emotional coping mechanisms are replaced or disrupted by the mood-altering substance. Elevated cortisol levels further aggravate the cognitive decline and stress state, creating a viciously self-perpetuating downward cycle.

The sum total effect is the HIJACKING OF THE BRAIN. As an organism, the addict is rendered helpless against his or her drug of choice and is vulnerable to injury or death.

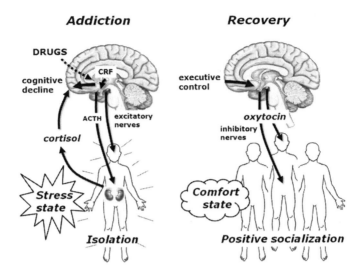

Recovery is characterized by a comfort state. There is decreased emotional reactivity to the everyday stresses of life. Nervous system balance is restored between inhibitory and excitatory systems. Our emotional control and maturity improves and, with these, improved decision-making and judgment. Other higher cognitive functions improve with time. As the illustration of brain imaging studies of meditation show (p. 224), areas activated by meditation (i.e., practicing non-reactivity to emotional stimulae) are those identical to those activated by cravings (p. 115) and deactivated in withdrawal and chronic mood-altering substance abuse (p. 120). Through positive empathetic socialization, there is elevation of the "comfort hormone" oxytocin, as well as other reward neurotransmitters (e.g., dopamine) responsible for "happiness and joy." Altruistic actions also bring joy and comfort. Natural rewards—such as food, exercise and sex—are rewarding once more and chosen over drug intoxication. The recovered individual is in control, content, relaxed, and calm. In recovery, as the authors of the *Big Book* so aptly put it, we become *"happy, joyous and free"* (p 133).

Closing Remarks

Addictive, mood-altering substances hijack our brains' core reward circuits, impairing our decision-making, motivation and ability to learn: Our emotional growth is stunted.

Both animals and humans grow best through enduring suffering and stress. We either adapt and strengthen, or suffer more. Sometimes we perish. Emotional growth can be achieved only through enduring hardship without the impedance of mood-altering substances.

Thankfully, through Twelve-Step recovery fellowships, we do not have to suffer alone. The joy of the positive empathetic support of the fellowship is a powerful substitute for mood-altering substances. The collective strength of our fellowship far exceeds that of any of its individual members. Our Creator made us so.

Ultimately, however, our individual recovery is measured by our personal emotional fortitude—'emotional sobriety'—and the depth and sincerity of our compassion for others.

Per the founding fathers of the Twelve-Steps: Our survival is incumbent on "unity, service, and recovery."

The recovery from addiction is a slow process, requiring sometimes-painful work. At times, we cannot see the progress that we have made. As slipping into addiction is often a slow and insidious process, so can be recovery.

In the rooms of Alcoholics Anonymous, I once heard a story about three men digging a ditch:

> *While on a leisurely stroll, a man came across three men digging a small, shallow ditch with shovels and picks. He asked the first man, "What are you doing?" and the man replied, "Digging a ditch." He asked the second man the same question, who said, "Making 12 dollars an hour." Finally, he asked the third man, who said, "Building a cathedral!"*
>
> *- Michael Levin*

~

The greatest danger for most of us is not that we aim too high and miss it—but aim too low and reach it.
~Michelangelo

Acknowledgements

First and foremost, I would like to thank my wife, Amy, for her love and enduring support. Similarly, I would like to thank my children, Joe, Giana, and Cara. The suffering they experienced as they watched their father killing himself with a bottle had to be unbelievable. I thank our nanny, Sherry, for her trustworthiness and dedication to our family. I thank my housekeeper, Julia, for keeping my place clean.

Thanks are due to my mother, Frances Teresi, who raised me right under extremely difficult circumstances. Thanks to my late father, Dr. Joseph Teresi, for good genes, providing a roof over my head, and the blessing of a good education. Thanks to my older brother, Joe, for being my best friend for 50 years and hands-down one of the smartest people I know. Thanks to my younger brother, Matt, one of the strongest men I know, and my sister, Ger, for being brave and stead-fast. Special thanks to Roy and Catherine Jacobson, my favorite mother-in-law, Betty Lutz, and late father-in-law, Lt. Col. Ed Lutz, (aviator and decorated WWII hero) for always loving me in tough times. Special thanks to Deborah Lutz and Karen Passow, who inspire me with their compassion and faith. Thanks to Uncle Bob Teresi for making me laugh and being the reigning patriarch of the Teresi family. May I also extend my gratitude to all my aunts, uncles and cousins from both sides of the family. You are beautiful people.

Thanks to my employers, friends and supporters in the radiology field (HC, WB, SL, JR, JS, and others) for never giving up on me and retaining my services in the field I love.

Special thanks must be extended to my counselors, Dr. Harry Haroutunian and Bob Newton of the Betty Ford Center, for cutting through my nonsense and giving me the tools to get out of the dark forest of my addiction. Of course, my gratitude extends to the entire staff of that treatment center for the kindness, courtesy and respect they showed me during my most vulnerable moments. My "inner child" thanks you.

I would like to thank all the researchers in the various fields referenced in this book. Your research and your observations are outstanding, and contributed to the saving of at least one life, mine. I simply connected the dots. I hope I did justice to your work. It is my hope that proceeds generated from this and other projects I have in mind will be directed to funding treatment scholarships and research.

Many thanks are also due to my sponsor, Neil M., my gandsponsor, Jim R., and all the members of my home group in California, Sunrise Sobriety, for unwavering empathy and compassion as I struggled with my addiction and my inability to cope with life on life's terms.

Finally, I posthumously thank Bill W. and Dr. Bob for starting the program of Alcoholics Anonymous and writing the *Big Book*. The organizations you spawned have saved the lives of millions from what once was called a "hopelessness condition of mind and body." I certainly hope I did justice to your work.

WARNING

I warn the reader *NOT* to ask your doctor or search the internet for oxytocin or related products. *Taking oxytocin can be dangerous.* I suspect other neurotransmitters also are involved in the "comfort response" and the relationships between neurotransmitters and neural circuits are very complex. I suspect oxytocin may be addictive itself. Clinical trials using oxytocin therapy, sponsored by the National Institute on Drug Addiction, are just beginning (NIDA, 2011).

I suspect there will be no "magic pill" or nasal mist that brings us the benefits of empathetic or affectionate relationships. If you want the comforting effects of empathetic social bonding or oxytocin, go to a meeting or call a friend and share your "stuff," snuggle with a loved one, get a massage, or listen to some soothing music. Meetings and massage (M&M Rx) are my personal favorites.

The above warning is consistent with a fundamental belief I have about medicine in general: *It is as much about what we know, as what we do not know. And we know only a little.*

Selected References

To save printing costs, all selected references (1,223 references, 97 pages) are available online at *hijackingthebrain.com*.

Index

Lightning Source UK Ltd.
Milton Keynes UK
UKOW050226080912

198648UK00001B/194/P